Food, Fun, n' Fitness:
Designing Healthy Lifestyles for Our Children

Designs for Healthy Lifestyles

Mary C. Friesz, Ph.D., R.D., C.D.E., L.D.N.

Food, Fun, n' Fitness: Designing Healthy Lifestyles for Our Children.
©2002 by Mary C. Friesz.

ISBN: 0-9715662-0-8

LCCN: 2002092935

Manufactured in the United States of America

This book is intended as an educational and informational resource. The publisher and author expressly disclaim any responsibility or liability in connection with the use of this book.

Certain terms mentioned in this book which are known or claimed to be trademarks or service marks have been capitalized. The author does not attest to the validity, accuracy, or completeness of this information. Use of a term in this book should not be regarded as affecting the validity of any trademark or service mark.

Cover design by Foster and Foster. Interior design by Nancy Gratton and by Publishing Professionals. Typeset by Publishing Professionals, New Port Richey, FL, Sylvia Hemmerly.

Dedication

To my son, Alexander,
whose health and happiness are my highest priorities.

Acknowledgments

As the saying goes, it takes a village to raise a child. Well, it also takes a small community to create a book. I'd like to thank my community, some of whom I've known all my life, others who have become new friends and colleagues in the course of making this book a reality. First, thanks to my family, who read my manuscript hundreds of times, offered advice and corrections, and never complained. Mom and Dad, Michele, and Kristina—I couldn't have done it without you! And, of course, I have to thank my son, Alexander—your patience and understanding while I worked on my book is what made this all possible.

Also adding their expertise and advice to the mix are Dr. David L. Bell, MD, MPH, who so graciously consented to write a foreword for this volume; and Dr. Beth Motzkin-Kava, a pediatric endocrinologist with whom I have had the pleasure to work. I would also like to thank my dear friend and colleague, Jacqueline King, MS, RD, CDE, FADA, for being one of the first to wade through the earliest manuscript notes and for sticking by me through the entire process. And thanks to Francis Berg, MS, LN, founder of the Healthy Weight Network, who has inspired so many to find a path to sound nutrition, exercise, and healthier lifestyles without resorting to the dangers of dieting.

Finally, I'd like to thank the team of professionals who worked so hard to make my dream of publishing this book come true. Thanks to my development editor, Nancy Gratton, who helped me put my thoughts into print. Thanks also to Sylvia Hemmerly and her team at Publishing Professionals, for turning the manuscript into a finished book. And thanks to George Foster, of Foster and Foster, Inc., for creating a cover design that so accurately captured my vision.

Foreword

It is a pleasure to be asked to say a few words about this timely book, which makes sense of the various societal, family and individual issues regarding our dietary and lifestyle habits in today's modern society. Writing this foreword is an honor for me, to be able to contribute to a valuable and well-balanced synthesis of current issues and strategies for parents to influence children and teenagers to maintain a healthy relationship with food, as well as to make healthy lifestyle choices.

As a pediatrician and adolescent medicine specialist, I see first hand many children and teenagers that are overweight and obese, struggling with maintaining a healthy weight, as well as suffering from cardiovascular risk factors and Type 2 diabetes as complications. I have also worked with teenagers suffering from anorexia nervosa and bulimia. There are so many messages about diets and dieting strategies present that it is difficult for the average or above average parent to make sense of it all for themselves and for their children. I am confident this book will serve as a useful reference for general information and practical strategies for addressing various lifestyle issues and problems for parents.

I applaud Dr. Mary for writing such an essential volume of valuable information!!

David L. Bell, M.D., M.P.H.
Assistant Professor of Pediatric and
Adolescent Medicine and Public Health
Columbia University, New York, New York

Table of Contents

Introduction

The development of a child is an amazing event. As a mom, I realize that I have been given a once in a lifetime opportunity to make a difference in someone's life. Someone who came into this world as an innocent infant in need of constant care, instant gratification, and a tremendous amount of attention is now my responsibility. As he grows, he comes to trust those who show him love and affection, and he looks to these individuals for the nurturing, protection and guidance he cannot provide for himself. I take my responsibility—to fulfill his needs—seriously.

With each day comes a new experience for both of us. Every day finds him discovering something he couldn't do the day before—a new action, attitude, or accomplishment. And every day I discover that my role as a parent goes much farther than providing my child with the mere essentials of life.

Like all parents, I bear the responsibility of assuring my child the best conditions for ultimate health and well-being; for providing sustenance for adequate growth; for providing clothing and shelter to shield from the elements outdoors; for protecting him from dangerous situations; and for teaching him the morals and values that he will need in order to become a compassionate, respectable human being. Unfortunately, as I grow in my recognition of these responsibilities, I have also grown ever more aware of how society seems to care less and less about them—blowing lots of hot air, but giving little real priority to family time, family values, and family health.

This is particularly clear when you consider how unresponsive today's society is to the needs of families who are now facing drastic changes in the way they live. The dramatic rise in the number of households where both parents must work; the sharp increase in single-parent households, the breakdown of the extended-family and the local community—all of these have put pressures on parents and children unknown in previous generations. But society as a whole seems unwilling or unable to provide much help. Instead, the focus seems to be on guaranteeing corporate profits and training our littlest citizens to become unquestioning consumers of every new fad and gimmick.

What's this got to do with nutrition and fitness, you might ask? To me, the answer is clear. With little outside support, parents today are facing an enormous challenge in trying to raise their children according to sound, healthy principles in the face of irresponsible advertising, an ever-expanding list of must-have (but not necessarily healthy) commodities, and a declining national commitment to the health and well-being of our children.

Children are our most precious resource—they are the joy of our present and the hope for our future. And nothing is more important to a growing child than the love and support of a close-knit family. But the truth is that we have become such a transient society that we often do not even know our neighbors. We live where we work, not where our families are, and we often do not get the chance to establish roots in our communities before it's time to move on again.

How does this affect our children? For one thing, they're losing a sense of connectedness with the world—not surprising in an age when computer games are their playmates and the television is their babysitter. But even more, it means that instead of getting their life-lessons from trusted adults, they depend more and more on the media to provide them with their image of the world.

As a single, working mom, I find this disturbing. As a professional in the field of nutrition, I find this actually frightening. The media, and the corporations who sponsor it, are not concerned with our children's well-being—they are interested in their bottom lines. And their priorities put them in direct confrontation with many of the principles that we, as parents, know we must uphold.

It is not in our children's best interests to abandon them to a life in which an addiction to technology, a sedentary lifestyle, and an over-reliance on junk-food are the order of the day. As parents, we must be committed to teaching them how to make choices that improve their chances for a healthy, happy life. And there's no time to waste! Childhood obesity and the diseases associated with it are on the rise, and eating disorders are reaching epidemic proportions among our nations young people.

That's why I wrote this book. It's my mission to educate parents about what they can do to ensure proper nutrition and healthy physical activity throughout childhood and the years of adolescence, in the face of all the media and social pressure to the contrary. I want to provide parents with a realistic approach to achieve these goals, so that our children do not grow up to be forever at the mercy of the latest advertising gimmick and food-and-fitness fad.

My interest in these issues comes from a very personal source. I suffered from obesity as a child, and although I eventually succeeded in overcoming that devastating condition, I found myself battling eating disorders during my teen and young adult years. These experiences led me to a career in nutrition and fitness, where I came to more deeply understand the wide range of factors that lead to these conditions in children. I became powerfully committed to working towards a future where our children can grow up well-nourished, fit, and happy, and out of this commitment I developed a program that I call Designs for Healthy Lifestyles.

A design for a healthy lifestyle is one in which children and adults can work together to promote good nutrition and fitness, thus preventing childhood obesity and the health problems associated with excess weight, both during childhood and later on, as adults. It is one in which parents can work with an already at-risk or obese child to work toward a healthy weight without triggering an obsession with weight that can lead to eating disorders. Most of all, it is one that promotes strengthened relationship bonds within families, helping every member to realize the healthiest, happiest lifestyle possible.

But I am aware that it isn't easy to fly in the face of all the pressures of modern living and to make the kind of changes required in order to get started on a healthy lifestyle. It requires challenging traditional assumptions about food, family, and fitness, and sometimes it means making some pretty basic changes in the way we go about our day-to-day lives. Still, the goal—the health of our children—is so important that I believe most parents will be willing to make the attempt. With this book, I hope to help you to take the first steps in designing the healthiest possible lifestyle for you, your family, and, most of all, for your children.

Let's get started!

Part One

Who's Raising Our Kids?

An Overview on Healthy Living

1

$\mathcal{I}$'m certain that we can all agree on at least one thing: we want our children to live healthy and happy lives. As a professional in the field of nutrition, I know that healthy living starts with healthy eating. But too often, and for lots of different reasons, we have trouble figuring out just what healthy eating is. Was it always like this?

In a word, no. Lifestyles have changed over the years, and some of these changes have had a definite, detrimental effect on how we view nutrition. To understand where we are—to define our present-day ground-zero in the fight for our children's health—it may be useful to take a closer look at where we came from, and how our lives have changed. So walk with me down memory lane, to see what life was like before the dawn of our current high-stress, high-tech, high-speed era.

TRAVELING BACK IN TIME

Years ago our food supply was quite different than it is today. Until as recently as the 1940s, agriculture was a huge part of the economy, and the foods were mostly grown on family farms, sold fresh- picked within the regions in which they were grown, relatively inexpensive, and largely unprocessed. What we ate at a given time was determined by seasonal availability, except for those items—mostly vegetables and legumes—that might be preserved and stored for later use. These preserves were the early version of "convenience

3

foods," but they bore little relation to the "convenience" and "fast" foods we know today.

Cooking practices were different back then, too. Fats were often added in the preparation of a meal, as a means of increasing the caloric value of the food, for lots of calories were needed to sustain people in their daily activities. After all, the average daily expenditure of physical energy in an agricultural, or even industrial, society was very high. This is why many of our traditional family recipes are high in starch and laden with fat—think of the oil customarily used in Spanish rice and bean recipes, the reliance on sour cream and noodles in the cuisines of Eastern Europe, the pasta and olive oil of Italian cookery, and the coconut milk and rice that typifies many traditional Caribbean recipes.

These meals made sense back then, because the average person's lifestyle was one of constant activity. On the farms, work consisted of such strenuous tasks as plowing the fields, churning butter, and collecting firewood. Today's conveniences were nonexistent, and even in the 1940s were still relatively rare—doing the laundry meant *really* scrubbing the clothes, often by hand; housework involved getting down on the floor with a wire brush and a bucket of soapy water; and, outside of the major cities and towns, marketing could well involve a walk of a mile or more, and a return trip carrying your purchases, because automobiles had not yet become a standard in most households.

Playtime for children was different then, too. Television didn't take over the average family home until the mid-1950s, so play meant *active* play—running around, climbing trees, swimming in the local pond, riding bicycles, and participating in games that got kids moving: *Red Rover, Mother May I, Tag*, and so on. Kids got neighborhood teams together for stickball, baseball, and football. And at the end of the day, they generally went to bed truly tired. The upshot of it all is that generations of the past were able to eat more calories because their active lifestyles required the excess energy as fuel. They burned those calories off each day, without ever even having to think much about it. But that's no longer true!

FAST-FORWARD TO THE PRESENT

Modern life is very different from what even our parents' generation knew. By the 1950s, the agricultural society had finally given way to an economy based on service and manufacturing, which meant that regular, daily physical activity was becoming less and less a part of people's lives. By the mid-1950s, as suburbs replaced formerly rural communities, the automobile had taken over the land, and at about the same time television had begun what would become a near-total take-over of the average family's living room (although it would be another decade before it truly "ruled the roost").

Meanwhile, healthy, fresh foods became less readily available: large acres of land once home to active farming were converted to suburbs, housing complexes, strip malls, and parking lots. Each year, less produce was grown and sold locally, and more imported foods turned up in our supermarkets. Prices of fresh fruits and veggies escalated, in part because of increased transportation costs, in part because it was easier for the producers to store and ship processed foods. The result: fresh, healthy food often cost more than processed, packaged foods.

By the 1960s, the way we lived had been radically transformed. Why walk when you can drive? Why go to the trouble of getting a group of kids together for a baseball game when you can keep them entertained with Saturday morning cartoons? Why prepare your own preserves from fresh ingredients when you can take a trip to the grocery store and stock up on canned goods? We became a much more sedentary society, and the changes didn't stop there.

By the 1970s, the cost of living had made it almost impossible for families to survive on one pay check. Fortunately, at the same time, there were increasing employment opportunities available to women, and two-income households became more common. But these changes meant more than just an increase in household income—they also meant that people had far less *time* for home activities. Here's something to think about: more than 25 percent of America's children are being raised by au pairs, in day care, or are enrolled in pre-schools.

And the entrepreneurs were quick to spot the trend. Labor-saving devices started appearing all over the place. In the 1950s and 1960s, the questions were: Why scrub your floors, when you can spritz some liquid on it and clean and wax it all at once. Why toil over a tub full of soapy water and dirty clothes, when you can install a machine that will let you get the job done at the push of a button? The physical energy we needed to expend to get through the day was dramatically reduced. And today it's reduced even further—especially for our children. Why ride your bike when you can slalom down a bicycle-racing course in virtual reality? Why get into a game of baseball, football, or basketball in the real world, when you can hook up your Sony or Sega and play a virtual game featuring sports celebrities? And, Mom, why "slave over a hot stove" when you can pick up a quickie, pre-made meal at the local fast-food store or in the supermarket freezer case?

Don't get me wrong, I am not against technology. It has opened a myriad of new avenues and opportunities—freeing us from the drudgery of many daily tasks and, with the advent of computers, enabling us to visit new worlds, keep abreast of current events, and stay in touch with loved ones near and far, all with a simple click of a mouse. BUT it does have its disadvantages, too—disadvantages that negatively affect our lifestyles, our activity levels, the quality of the foods we eat, and ultimately our health.

What About Today?

Here's a scary thought: In the November 13, 2000 issue of *Time* magazine, Michael Jacobson, co-founder of the Center for Science in the Public Interest, told reporter Margot Roosevelt that "our society encourages sloth and gluttony. Obesity and related illnesses, such as diabetes, heart disease, and cancer, cause as many deaths as tobacco." As a professional in the field of diet and nutrition, I know that Jacobson is not exaggerating the case. I know, for instance, that American kids watch an average of 3.5 to 4 hours of TV a day—and that many watch much more, because the TV has become the babysitter of first-resort in many homes.

And I know—because I see it in my practice all the time—there's been a tremendous decrease in available physical activities for kids, both at home and in school. With more households where both parents work full time, many kids come home to empty houses—killing time watching TV, playing computer or video games, and snacking on junk food. Going outside to play after school just doesn't happen that much anymore, because our neighborhoods are not as friendly or as safe as they once were.

Even at school, activity is on the decline. School funding is a real problem, and unfortunately, physical education is usually one of the first classes to be eliminated. Gone are the days of mandatory gym class. When I was in school, we had gym daily and if you failed in gym, you failed for the year, regardless of your grades. But now, in many public schools, kids are lucky to get physical education for a couple of weeks a year!

And while we're on the subject of schools—don't think your children are safe from the junk food epidemic even there! The National School Lunch Program was initially intended to provide one-third of the nutritional recommended daily allowance (RDA) to children who normally would not have access to healthy meals. When the breakfast program was inaugurated, it was intended to provide another one-third of the RDA as well. But look what has happened to those early, well-intended programs! The average school meal is high in fat and calories, largely because it is based on USDA subsidies and has become the dumping-ground for surplus of lower-quality goods that don't make the grade for commercial sale. Fresh produce is rarely available. And cost-cutting doesn't stop there: Most of us remember the great "ketchup is a vegetable" debate of the 1980s when, in the interests of cost-cutting, the government suggested that this no-food-value condiment could count as a vegetable portion in school lunch planning!

More recently, schools have responded to shrinking budgets by allowing companies to place soda and snack vending machines in our schools. Soda companies and others actively bid to gain exclusive vending-machine placement rights in individual schools, offering kickbacks of 25 to 50 percent of the sales (school officials frequently refer to these as "fund raisers"), and our revenue-starved school systems grab these opportunities for a little extra cash in the budget. The result: schools are sending hypocritical messages to our kids. Even though they're supposed to be teaching the importance of health in the classroom, they're providing high-profile marketing space for everything from Coke and Pepsi to McNuggets and Whopper Juniors! Even if our schools managed to improve on the standard school lunch fare tomorrow, how could they compete for our children's lunch money when they have to compete with vending machines that dispense candy and colas or, in a more recent and disturbing trend, with the in-school kiosks run by companies like McDonald's, Burger King, and Taco Bell?

A MULTIFACETED PROBLEM

Ironically, our nation is facing a nutrition and fitness crisis at a time when we seem to be more health-conscious than ever before. Our lawmakers are constantly pushing for "better health care" and we, as a society, spend mega-millions of dollars each year on products touted as promoting "health and longevity." Billions are spent annually on nutritional supplements, herbal remedies, and alternative health therapies with the hope of finding the fountain of youth. Yet obesity, eating disorders, and other nutritionally related illnesses are on the rise throughout all segments of society, and most particularly among our youth.

How did this happen? Largely because of short-sighted, quick-fix policies and a poor understanding of the root causes of poor nutrition. We haven't come to grips with the variety of factors that influence the way we eat and the food choices we make for ourselves and our children. My mission, to which I have dedicated my professional life, is to change this state of affairs. I am convinced that, once we understand just what goes into our nutritional decision-making, we will all be better prepared to make the necessary changes—for the sake of our children's health!

So, just what are these all important, influential factors that have fed into the rise in obesity and other nutrition-related health issues, especially among our children? They can be broken down into three distinct categories:

1. Family and Lifestyle Issues: These include the social and cultural factors that underlie our basic understanding of what constitutes "good" foods and "proper" meals; the role played by our emotions and body-image attitudes in deciding when, what, and how much to eat; and the constraints that today's fast-paced lifestyles place upon our day-to-day nutritional choices and our commitment to healthy activity.

2. Media and Marketing Issues: These include the all-pervasive role of advertising in shaping our attitudes toward food; the conflict between food-production-for-profit versus food-consumption-for-health; and the way that you—and your children—have become the battleground for competing commercial enter-

prises that view our households as market-shares in the competition for revenues.

3. The March of Technology: This refers to the way that our patterns of activity have steadily evolved over the past several decades, and the way that these changes have altered our nutritional needs from those of generations past. Most particularly, it refers to the fact that, while our activity patterns have changed radically, our consumption patterns have not adequately responded to these changes.

In the next three chapters we'll take a close look at each of these factors, but for now let's get in a quick overview of them, one-by-one.

Family Values And Lifestyle Issues

Food is not, and probably never has been, viewed purely as a means of relieving hunger. It is associated with all sorts of social and cultural issues. Just think about it: there is no social event that isn't somehow associated with food. Life events like weddings and funerals are traditionally marked with a special meal. The same is true for holidays: what would Thanksgiving be without a turkey? Christmas without a ham? Passover without its traditional ritual meals? Even non-eating has a ritual food component: Lenten fasting is followed by the traditional Easter feast. The close of Yom Kippur and Ramadan are similarly marked.

And it's not just the big, ritual occasions that are associated with food. Going to a movie? You immediately think of a big bucket of popcorn drenched with butter (or butter-substitute). A sports event? Gotta run to the concession stand for hot dogs and soda or beer, right? How about the amusement park or the annual county fair? Fast-food galore, perhaps best typified by colorful puffs of cotton candy on a stick!

And we associate food with other things as well. We all have our own idea of what constitutes "comfort foods"—the foods that make us feel better when we're feeling low. And we associate food with particular times, regardless of whether or not we're hungry. At noon, it's lunchtime! After school means after-school snacks! And too many of us eat out of boredom, in response to stress, or just because it's *there* (after all, weren't we all taught to "clean our plates" as children?).

We'll probably never think of food solely as fuel (and, in fact, life would seem a little sad if we did). But that's no reason to stay hooked on negative eating habits. What we need to do is teach ourselves—and, most importantly, our children—to tune into our bodies, to distinguish between "mind hunger" and true hunger, and to eat until we're satisfied and stop when we've had enough.

But it's not just how we think about food that affects our children's eating habits and attitudes toward health and fitness. Body-image, peer-pressure, and problems of self-esteem play a big part in this as well. In Chapter 2 you'll learn a lot more about this, and we'll begin to look at ways in which you can help your children develop healthier attitudes about what foods they eat.

Media and Marketing Issues

Let's get one thing clear right now: food producers aren't in the business out of concern for your health. The American food industry is big business—billion-dollar big business—and its primary goal is to make a profit—which can only be done if you, and millions of others like you, can be coerced to buy its products. That means marketing, and marketing *aggressively!* Product placement in movies (notice the hero in the film carefully holding that can of brand-name soda with the label toward the camera?), promotional tie-ins (all those tiny collectible toys packed in with your "kiddie meal" at the local fast-food restaurant), and contests (turn in 6 lucky bottle caps and win a prize! collect 5 proof-of- purchase seals from the giant-sized box of a certain sugary cereal and you can win a cheap plastic spoon that *talks!*) are all ways that the industry tries to get you to buy (or your kids to demand) their product.

And there are more pernicious marketing ploys out there, too. There are even companies that have established special divisions devoted expressly to marketing to kids! A case in point is Griffin Bacal, Inc., which puts out a special newsletter called *Kidcurrents: Perspectives on Youth Marketing.* This should be no surprise. Companies know that kids are important to both short- and long-term sales. Not only do kids represent a pretty well-funded market in their own right, they also influence how their parents spend their food dollars, clamoring for the latest heavily advertised product, begging for a complete set of collectible toys "included in every kiddie meal." And the companies know if they get a child's loyalty early in life, that child will probably stay with the product well into adulthood!

Even worse is how marketing has invaded our schools!! I've already mentioned the influx of vending machines, but there have been more disturbing developments going on right under the noses of our teachers and school boards. For example, in 1990, Frimedia, Inc. began offering free audio-visual equipment to our cash-strapped public schools, with the requirement that partici- pating schools commit to incorporating their educational pro- gram, called Channel One, in the daily lesson plan. Sounds pretty altruistic, doesn't it? Lots of schools thought so—the program is now a regular part of the curriculum in more than 12,000 schools around the country. But there's a big catch to this "gift": for every 10 minutes of news or current events carried on Channel One, there are 2 minutes of pure advertising, touting the products of Coca Cola, Pepsi, M&M/Mars, McDonald's, Burger King, and much, much more! And there are corporately sponsored educa- tional aids—workbooks and textbooks—that prominently feature the sponsors' products. For example, one workbook explicitly uses M&Ms and Tootsie Rolls as "counters" to teach basic math! Other companies offer free book covers to the schools, with their corpo- rate logo prominently featured, of course—so our kids become walking billboards for their products!

It seems almost impossible to avoid the marketing pressures, doesn't it? But being forewarned is being fore-armed—in Chap- ter 3 you'll learn more about the influence of media and marketing on food choices, and how to counteract them.

The March of Technology

Technological changes have affected our ideas about health, food, and fitness in a number of ways. First and foremost, we've seen a steady reduction in the sheer physical activity required to accom- plish our day-to-day tasks: labor-saving devices have reduced the drudgery—and the caloric consumption—of many of our chores. As cars became an everyday necessity instead of a luxury reserved for the rich, we became a nation of riders, not walkers. Elevators whisk us upward, relieving us of the necessity of climbing stairs. Life has become a lot less physically demanding than it was just a few decades ago. And while I'm all for the convenience of these devices, I'm less thrilled with the fact that we've paid so little attention to finding new physical outlets for our energy.

What's scariest of all is how technology has reconfigured the landscape of childhood. Labor-saving devices are one thing, play-substitutes are another thing entirely. Yet that's what we've gotten as television, computers, and video games have taken over our children's leisure time. Kids spend hours parked in front of the television—which is bad on two counts: first, because there's little interactivity involved (the old days of *Romper Room*, with its regular 10-minute feature of exercises, is long gone—today's programs largely promote passive watching); second, because every program is loaded with commercials, many of which aggressively tout the virtues of this fast-food joint, or that high-sugar cereal.

And when our kids aren't watching TV, they're probably hooked up to a video game. But successfully maneuvering your Mario Brother, Sonic the Hedgehog, or Lara Croft through the mazes on the screen doesn't provide any real exercise for anybody except the cartoon characters who are doing all the work! On the school playground, it's not unusual these days to see the monkey- bars, ball-fields, and swing sets standing empty, while clusters of kids spend their recess period punching the keys of their hand-held video games instead—and that's if they even get an outdoor recess at all (with the increasing dangers in today's schools, many have opted for keeping the kids indoors for the entire school day).

Even more subtly, our increased reliance on technology has had a further effect on our children's physical well-being. The attraction of the electronic universe, in video games and on the Internet, has been a powerful force in causing a great deal of isolation—not just for kids but for all of us. We get the semblance of community with our on-line chat rooms, e-mail, and instant messaging, but little true human contact. That breaks down our ability—and even our desire—for regular participation in "real-time" relationships. According to Edward M. Hallowell, M.D., a psychiatrist on the faculty at Harvard Medical School, "Connectedness (that is, staying connected with family and friends) is as much a protective factor—probably more—than lowering your blood pressure, losing weight, quitting smoking, or wearing your seat belt."

And a nine-year study of 7,000 people in Alameda, California, reinforced Dr. Hallowell's findings. In the December 2000 issue of *Prevention* magazine, reporter Ellen Michaud revealed that those with the fewest connections to family and friends were three times more likely to die over the lifetime of the study than those who had the most such connections, even though members of the latter group smoked, drank, or indulged in a high-fat diet! No one knows exactly *how* it works, but the evidence clearly indicates that human connectedness seems to enhance the immune system and lower both blood pressure and heart rates.

In Chapter 4 we'll explore these and other technologically related issues and how they have a direct impact upon your child's health and well-being—particularly with regard to their effect upon attitudes about nutrition and activity. But more than just presenting a catalog of the problems, I'll also provide you with ways to overcome them.

CREATING A NEW DESIGN FOR HEALTHY LIVING

With all these factors working against us, what can parents do to fight the trend toward bad nutrition, reduced activity, and generally declining health standards for our children? It may seem hopeless, but I'm here to tell you that it's not. Like you, I'm faced with the daily pressures to give in to fast-food and to take so-called short-cuts—as a single Mom and full-time, working parent, it sometimes seems easier to just "go with the flow." But I have had two powerful reasons to find a better way. First, my personal experience has taught me that the price-tag is just too high: I personally suffered, physically and emotionally, from obesity in my childhood, and during adolescence I had first-hand experience with two truly dangerous eating disorders. I overcame all of these problems, but in doing so I learned just how desperately difficult it is to beat them once they've become established in a child's life. And second, my professional training has taught me that the "short cuts" are illusory—it's really not all that difficult to establish, and maintain, a healthy lifestyle for our children, even in the face of all of today's many pressures. Read on, and I'll share with you the insights I've derived from a lifetime dedicated to healthy living—for the health of our children!

Family Values and Lifestyles

2

$\mathcal{M}$any factors contribute to whether or not you and your children practice healthy eating and fitness habits. Some of these factors are obvious: the foods you choose to eat and the amount of exercise you build into your day-to-day life, for example, are lifestyle choices that are clearly connected to your general level of wellness. But other factors are less obvious—like the assumptions that we make about nutrition and exercise that we never really question, and that we often pass along to our children, without even thinking about them. In this chapter we'll take a look at some of those unquestioned values and assumptions that may be influencing our choices. I believe that after reading this chapter you'll be better prepared to question some of these assumptions in the future—and you'll be able to break free of them.

Questioning Assumptions

Each of us has inherited certain ideas and beliefs that influence our choices when it comes to food and nutrition. As you learned in Chapter 1, some of these ideas have their roots in practices that date back to a time and a culture that no longer apply. Thus, depending upon your particular cultural and ethnic background, you may feel that a meal simply isn't a meal unless it includes meat, or rice, or a pasta dish—or concludes with a rich, gooey dessert. Or you may feel that the day truly doesn't begin until you've had a huge breakfast including bacon, eggs, and bread. But these culturally and ethnically conditioned attitudes toward food are only the tip of the iceberg. There are many other "family values" and lifestyle factors that intrude on the nutrition and fitness choices we make for ourselves and for our children. And, by failing to examine some of these values, we run the risk of passing along some unhealthy ideas along to our kids.

For example, who would have thought that the growth of suburban communities and changes in urban housing construction could have an impact on the nutritional health and physical fitness of our kids? But that's just what has happened. Here's how.

A Community of Strangers

Years ago, kids were greatly influenced by the people of their local community, which generally included their extended families. Parents and siblings, aunts and uncles, cousins, teachers, and neighbors all had more direct involvement in the way our kids grew up. For example, when I was a kid, I grew up in a good, old-fashioned neighborhood, where everyone knew everyone and all the adults would watch out for each other's children and property. Kids could roam the neighborhood, feeling free and unsupervised, but there was always an adult around—often a relative—to keep a watchful eye out for their safety. And for a long time this was true even in the cities—there was always somebody looking out of an apartment window or sitting on the stoop, watching the street traffic and, incidentally, keeping an eye on what the kids were up to.

Now, however, things have changed dramatically. People are so mobile that neighbors often go for years without knowing the people who live next door! After all, why bother to get to know your neighbors if the odds are that they'll be moving away within a year or two? And in the cities, where old brownstones and 5-story walk-ups have been replaced by gigantic apartment buildings, the change is even more obvious. Back in the late 1980s, when I lived in a high rise in Manhattan, people would get onto the elevator and, even though they knew full well that all the other passengers lived in the same building (community), they never spoke to one another—some would look at the floor while the others looked at the ceiling—rarely did anyone ever make eye contact!

Today's society is so transient that the majority of our communities are no longer as closely knit as they once were. Young adults choose to set up their own households according to where they work, not where the rest of their family lives, so today's communities are, in large part, communities of strangers—*not* people you can count on to watch out for your kids during your absence. Whether you live in a high-income, exclusive community or a low-income housing development, your fears are the same: no one is free from the fear of crime or random violence.

For a while, recently, it looked as if this trend was reversing itself. In the aftermath of the terrible events of September 11, 2001, it looked as if people were rediscovering a sense of community and neighborliness. But as time goes on and the memory recedes, and the stress of day-to-day living reasserts itself, we seem to be slipping right back into our isolated ways.

How does this impact upon the nutritional health and fitness of our children? Gone are the days when we could feel safe even when our children were out of our sight. Lacking a neighborhood community to rely upon, we no longer dare to allow our children to play outside without parental supervision. But as more and more households find it difficult to survive on a single income, parental supervision is increasingly hard to provide and, as a result, many kids today are "latch-key kids," told to go straight home after school and stay in the house, for safety reasons. What do they *do*? Watch TV, play video games, hop onto the Internet—and snack!

The unexpected consequence of these changes has been that playtime has shifted from the exercise afforded by a good, long bike-ride, climbing trees, or just plain running around, to mashing video-game controller buttons or clicking a mouse! And there's the refrigerator and kitchen cabinets temptingly near by, full of processed, high fat, sugary snacks!

A New Breed of Role Models

The reduction of sheer physical exercise for kids is not the only devastating effect of our new "communities of strangers." With the decreased presence of adults actively involved in their lives and their communities, it should come as no surprise that children are no longer greatly influenced by what those adults think is best. Instead, children are now influenced more by what they watch on

TV, read, and see on the Internet, and by their music, video games, and peers. If they have real-life adult influences, they're likely to be childcare workers or teachers. And while some of these influences may be positive, or at least benign—good teachers, good books, caring childcare professionals, for example—others are not. After all, the bulk of the "entertainment" available to kids on TV, video and, increasingly, on the Internet, is motivated by commercial interests, not sound principles of child-rearing.

The Disappearing Parents

What are the root causes of the decline in parental influence over our kids' values? One major contributing factor is the rise in two-income households, a trend that began as early as the 1970s. Another is the rise in single-parent households. Divorce statistics increased dramatically throughout the 1970s and 1980s and, although there has been a heartening trend to fewer divorces starting in the 1990s, the number of households headed by single parents remains high. Both of these facts of modern life have meant that the parental presence in children's lives has been reduced—and even when parents are home from their jobs, they're often tired enough to willingly let the TV or video games amuse the kids.

When I was a kid, any time I was home from school, Mom was there too. And at least for the evening meal—and usually breakfast, too—the whole family ate together. And on Sundays, after church, we *always* ate as a family—either at home or with relatives. It was unthinkable that we'd take our meals separately, or eat while parked in front of the television. So we always had at least one time every day when everybody "checked in" with one another and shared information about what we'd been doing at school or work. And after dinner, we kids would play outside if the weather was good and it wasn't too dark out. Watching TV was a family affair—so my parents always knew what we kids were watching.

Today, however, home-cooked meals are becoming rare, and it's not uncommon for families to go all week without actually sitting around the table, all together for a meal. This means that meals have become something of a "grab and go" affair, but it also means that there are fewer opportunities for parents to interact with their children.

And when it comes to the TV, things have changed even more dramatically. Did you know that about 35 percent of all Americans, between the ages of 2 and 7 have TV's in their own rooms? And that the number rises to a whopping 65 percent for children between the ages of 8 and 18? Watching TV is no longer a form of family entertainment for most households—it's a solitary pursuit.

But if everybody is retreating to their own rooms to watch TV, how is a parent supposed to keep track of the kinds of influences the programming is having on their kids? Now add in the sheer number of hours most kids are spending glued to the tube—an average of 24 hours per week. The programs are bad enough, sometimes, but according to Dr. Alvin Poussaint and Susan Linn, Ed.D., they're also watching more than 576 commercials each week. That's more than 20,000 commercials each year—and that's only the advertising they're exposed to on television! That's not counting magazines, newspapers, billboards, radios . . . you get the picture. (See their article, "Surviving Television Advertising," on the Family Education Network Website: familyeducation.com.) We owe it to our kids to be better informed about just what it is they're watching!

CULTURE CLASHES

Even when the family does share mealtimes, we don't necessarily make the wisest food choices when it comes to nutrition— for ourselves or for our kids. First of all, even we parents aren't immune to making mistakes based on incomplete information or unquestioned assumptions about healthy eating.

For example, lots of children who were born in the 1950s and 1960s grew up to love Wonder Bread sandwiches and chicken noodle soup from a can, as a typical cold-weather lunch. Not surprisingly, as adults they're likely to offer the same sorts of foods to their own kids. But today we know something that Moms back in the 50s and 60s weren't aware of: the refined flour in white bread lacks important nutrients, and the canned soups have TONS of salt. We'd be much better off to break with "tradition" and use whole grain breads for the sandwiches, while checking the labels for low-sodium soups.

Another time when we tend to carry on traditions that are no longer appropriate is at holiday meals. Most of us grew up with the idea that holidays meant having a huge dinner with lots of desserts to follow—and eating until we were too stuffed to move! Then, after the meal, we'd park ourselves in front of the TV to catch the holiday specials or the football game—not a good way to work off those calories!

Even more dangerous are the attitudes about dieting and fitness that we pass along to our kids without thinking. This is a problem that hits girls particularly hard, because they tend to adopt their mothers' attitudes about body image and weight issues. If you've internalized the "thin is in" myth, then you're probably going to pass some form of body-image neurosis along to your own children—with potentially devastating long-term results. Or if you're accustomed to using food for comfort (lots of people turn to food when they're feeling stressed or sad), your children are liable to do the same. In either case, they lose sight of the proper reason for eating—to provide the body with the fuel it needs. They lose the ability to tune in and listen to their bodies and to distinguish between emotional hunger and true, physical hunger.

LIFE IN THE FAST LANE

Today's fast-paced lifestyle has had another unexpected consequence on our attitudes about food. We—and especially our kids—have lost the ability to tune in to our bodies' hunger signals. We eat because it's "time"—lunch time, snack time—or because something looks and smells good, or just because it's *there*, even when we aren't really hungry. For example, in some of our public schools, there are so many kids that the administration has to schedule "lunch-time" in shifts, because the lunch room can't handle them all at once. In some really overcrowded schools, "lunch" can be as early as 10:30 a.m.! Somehow we need to teach our children to tune in and listen to their bodies, and to distinguish mind-hunger ("gee, I'd like a snack right about now") from true body hunger—that hollow, belly-growling, empty feeling. Eating for reasons aside from actual body hunger is not a healthy habit to establish. Sure an occasional bite of something just because it looks or smells good won't have long-term effects, but it will if it becomes a frequent, unnoticed habit.

Another detrimental effect of our fast-paced lifestyle is that we are all much more prone to eating "on the run"—which too often means eating highly processed, fat and sugar-laden convenience foods. Sugar-filled toaster pastries are treated as a substitute for a good breakfast; and school lunch periods are as short as half an hour—half of which is used up just *getting* the food. Instead of making a sit-down, home-cooked dinner, over-burdened parents find it easier to pick up a pizza or take the kids to the local fast-food joint.

Unfortunately, the effect of these decisions lasts well beyond the moment. Not only are these kinds of meals often nutritionally lacking—they also set a pattern that may haunt your kids later in life. Foods that are given early on often dictate the taste preferences our kids develop. If we start feeding our kids highly sweetened or fatty foods, we'll set them up for wanting these foods all the time. That's a shame, when it's just as easy to introduce healthier foods —like whole grains, veggies, and fresh fruits—instead.

You'll probably never get a child to skip junk foods entirely, of course, because there's peer pressure to deal with, too. My son loves fresh fruits and veggies when he's at home because these are the foods he's grown up with. It's just that, when he's with friends his age—kids who poo-poo veggies—he's likely to make a show of not liking them. Still, when he's at home he eats them quite happily. A slip or two is natural—as long as the healthy-eating habit gets a solid start.

CHANGING ATTITUDES ABOUT FOOD

One little recognized factor that affects our food choices is the change that has taken place in what we define as food. That may sound strange, but think about it—in our grandmother's day, good food mostly meant fresh meats, fruits and vegetables in season, and home-baked—or at least fresh-baked—breads. In the 1940s and 1950s, however, our food supply began to change. America fell in love with all the new technologies and labor-saving innovations that started springing up. This is when the food processing industry really took off, and it's been going strong ever since.

The result: Many so-called "foods" on grocery shelves today wouldn't even have been considered edible a few generations ago! Did you ever try and decipher the labels of things like Froot Roll-Ups or Lunchables? These products are mainly chemicals that have been shaped and dyed to look like food! Other products may start out with real ingredients, but then they're shot full of chemicals and preservatives.

Why did this happen? Mostly to prolong "shelf life"—foods full of preservatives can be shipped longer distances and kept on the store shelves longer if they're loaded with preservatives, which means that the manufacturers lose less money. And chemicals and hormones can make a piece of fruit or meat look appetizing long after it would otherwise spoil.

But think about it—how could anything that sits on a shelf, with an expiration over a year away, be considered "good for you" food? The amount of preservatives and chemicals needed to keep it edible is astronomical. (I always say, the reason people are living longer these days is because of the preservatives in our food supply —they're "preserving" our insides too!)

Take a walk through any grocery store, and what do you see? Aisle after aisle of pre-packaged, prepared foods full of additives. They promise us convenience—one-dish dinners, "cooks in 5 minutes," "instant entrees"—but for all this convenience you're sacrificing nutritional quality. To find the *real* food you have to really look for it. Supermarkets place the staple goods and fresh produce around the edges of the store, in hopes that you'll have to go up and down the aisles (filled with the higher-priced, processed stuff) to get there. In a similar strategy, they put the unprocessed staples on the bottom shelves, hoping that the brightly packaged, chemical-laden products shelved at eye level will get your attention first.

THE HIGH COST OF CONVENIENCE

Our preoccupation with convenience is costly—both in terms of health and in money. Food is the second largest expense (after housing) that parents pay out for their children—it accounts for a full 15 to 20 percent of total child-rearing costs. And the reason the costs are so high is that we've gotten hooked on the false bargain of convenience foods. For example, those fast-food "Value Meal Deals" sound like a real bargain, right? Hey, back in the 1960s, McDonald's even used their low prices in their ads: "you'll get change back from your dollar." But when you realize that the nutritional value of such meals is so low, the average per-meal price of between $4 and $5 doesn't look like so much of a bargain anymore.

But, as a nation, we're not heading out to McDonald's for the occasional treat. In the 1980s, American families only ate 25 percent of their meals outside the home—now we're eating out a full 50 percent of the time. For families with young children, those dining-out experiences most frequently mean fast-food places, because they're so kid-friendly and because they are comparatively inexpensive.

And, hey, for an extra 69 cents you can "Super-Size" your order! Sounds like a real bargain for a budget-conscious family that wants to eat out, right? But take a look at what happens to your calories, fat, and salt consumption when you go for that bargain:

A Kid's Hamburger Value Meal Has:			
	Calories	**Fat (g)**	**Salt (mg)**
Hamburger	270	10	580
Cheeseburger	380	19	770
Small Fries	210	10	125
Small Hi-C	120	0	20
Skim Milk	80	1.5	115
Typical Adult "Value Meal"			
Big Mac	560	31	1070
Double Whopper w/Cheese	960	63	1420
Super Fries	540	26	350
Super Hi-C	350	0	60

Okay, now if you do the math, you'll find that a typical "kid's meal" with cheeseburger, small fries, and (let's pick the "healthy" drink option) a skim milk comes to 670 calories. Doesn't sound too bad at first, but look at where the calories come from! Every gram of fat is 9 calories, and the "kid's meal" contains 30.5 grams of fat. That means 274.5 calories—more than 30 percent of the meal

—comes from fat! And while we're doing the math, take a look at the sodium: 1,010 milligrams. That's half a teaspoon!

Now take a look at the "adult meal": Big Mac, Super-sized fries, and a super-sized Hi-C. Add up the calories and this poor soul gets a whopping 1,450 calories! That's only a little less than the total calorie allotment for a typical adult female FOR A WHOLE DAY! Now look at the amount that comes from fat: 57 grams, or 513 calories! That's like eating 5 tablespoons of pure lard! And the sodium is just as bad: a heaping 1,480 milligrams. That's like eating almost a teaspoon of salt!

Think you're better off ordering a Taco Salad? Think again. That'll give you 850 calories, of which 468 comes from fat, seasoned with 2,250 milligrams of sodium (a teaspoon of sodium is just 2,000 milligrams). Where's all that fat and salt coming from? Here's the surprise: the taco shell is the biggest offender. Ditch the shell and you'll cut the numbers, saving yourself 400 calories, 30 grams of fat (270 calories), and 260 milligrams of sodium. Now we're talking!

And it's not just the fast-food places that load you up with empty calories. Snack-food manufacturers do it too: the 1-ounce snack-sized bag of chips have become 1.5 to 3 ounce "grab bags," giving you double and triple the calories, fat, sugar, and salt in the process; candy bars have been "king-sized;" and the standard 8-ounce serving of a soft drink has *really* grown, to 32-ounce "Big Gulps" and even 64 ounce "Super Big Gulps"!

Most family-oriented restaurants try to compete with the fast-food establishments by offering very large portions. Unfortunately, this leads to another problem: we've been taught to "clean our plates" and eat everything we're served, even when it's more than we really want—otherwise we're afraid we won't "get our money's worth." But notice that the large servings tend to be potato-, rice-, and pasta-based. These are very inexpensive staples, so the restaurants can afford to be generous in their portions, giving you the illusion of getting a good meal deal. It's no big bargain! In fact, if you eat everything they serve you, you're basically just paying to kill yourself!

SCHOOL DAZE

Finally, our society's changing values and our modern life-styles have had an impact—not always for the better—on the resources that parents once trusted to help reinforce their efforts in behalf of their children's well-being. I'm talking about the educational system here.

It used to be that parents counted on their children's schools to promote a message of healthy living, along with teaching our kids readin', writin', and 'rithmetic. The school lunch programs were designed to provide a hot, balanced meal for a reasonable fee, and every school considered some sort of physical education an essential part of every school day. In the 1960s, there was even a President's Council on Physical Fitness, which promoted formal athletics and even established competency guidelines for each stage of a child's growth. That council still exists—now it's called the President's Council on Physical Fitness and Sports—but schools rarely participate in it anymore!!

What caused the change? In the 1970s, voters started rebelling against property tax rates (most communities fund their public schools through the property tax), so school budgets started shrinking. And since then, politicians have been quick to seize the anti-tax movement to slash programs across the board—with education often being the first to get cut. That meant that schools had to start looking for ways to economize, and physical education—at least in the grade schools—was usually one of the first programs to suffer.

Clearly, today's educational system is much too political for its own good. Politicians appear to be more interested in arguing over standardized tests than they are about the conditions in our schools and the effect that those conditions can have on our children's ability to learn. Educators used to recognize the importance of the mind-body link—in fact, one of the principle goals of education was to foster "*mens sana in corpore sano*" (a sound mind in a sound body). And child development experts still know this to be true. Here's what Robert J. Doman Jr., of the American Academy of Child Development, had to say on the subject, in his 1986 article, published in the *Journal of the National Academy of Child Development*, "The Learning Environment":

> Children learn as a result of the input which their brain receives from their senses. We may be able to make a child stay in one place for an extended period of time (duration)

while we go over material (frequency) but the child has control over the intensity of the input. The child can be turned on or turned off. If turned on, he learns rapidly; if turned off, learning may never occur.

Fixing Food Service in School

While politicians argue over standardized testing, we're ignoring the fact that our children need a safe, creative, and enjoyable atmosphere in which to learn. And we appear to have completely given up on training their bodies as well as their minds. Instead, schools seem to have become training grounds for the production of a new generation of little consumers—and much of what they promote is detrimental to healthy living: allowing vending machines in the cafeterias and commercial-saturated "educational television" in the classrooms, as well as using brand-name candies as "teaching aids"!

This, too, has occurred because of changes in our values and lifestyles. We've become accustomed to turning over the day-to-day responsibility for our kids to the schools because our over-extended lives seemed to demand it. But we haven't compensated for this decision by becoming active after-hours in the workings of our local schools or our school boards. Without our active participation, the decisions of budget-cutters and politicians will go unchallenged.

And I honestly believe that nutrition and fitness are crucial areas in which parents can get involved. The importance of nutrition on academic performance is well known by professionals in the field. And taking charge at breakfast time is one way to make a big difference.

For example, forget about how all the ads stress convenience foods for breakfast. A toaster pastry and a glass of juice is basically just a high-sugar, total-carbohydrate meal—what I call a "fortified sugar rush." It will only keep a kid fueled for about an hour! On the other hand, a breakfast consisting of whole-grain cereal, a banana, and milk, with its complex carbohydrates, would keep them going for about 2 hours. For even more staying power, try an egg served with toast or an English muffin topped with peanut butter and fruit spread: it'll provide fuel for a full 4 to 5 hours! That's because the protein takes longer to digest, keeping them feeling satiated longer.

Obviously, breakfast with protein is the best bet, but the whole-grain cereal is still much better than that sticky, sugary toaster pastry. And there are other options, too: how about grilled cheese on toast? Or low-fat yogurt with granola? Or a quick sandwich of cream cheese and fruit spread? They're all options that will give your children a better start on their school day!

Nutritionists know that kids who start the day without breakfast are likely to have problems paying attention in class, and that sugary cereals and pastries or high-fat snacks give children a burst of energy that is quickly followed by a drastic plummet, leaving kids too tired to learn. Their blood is busy racing to the stomach to aid in digestion, leaving less for the brain to use. On the other hand, kids who get a good breakfast get a longer-lasting boost from the meal, have a more stable energy level, and come closer to meeting their overall nutrient needs for the day, including their need for calcium and iron, thanks to the fortified cereals and milk.

Parents can start paying attention to the food programs and policies in their children's schools. We can press to have junk-food and soda vending machines removed from school grounds. We can insist on reviewing the weekly school-lunch menus. You might be shocked by what you find: according to a report by the American School Foodservice Association, published in the October 20, 2000, issue of *Time for Kids*, the top 5 school lunch foods are:

1. Pizza
2. Chocolate chip cookies
3. Corn
4. French fries
5. Chicken nuggets

Most of these don't even qualify as a full meal—and *really*, chocolate chip cookies as a *lunch!?*

And while we're on the subject of food in the schools, here's something else you may not be aware of. Lots of teachers will give out candy as "prizes" for a correct answer or a job well done. By doing this, they're teaching kids a couple of things that just aren't healthy over the long term. For one thing, they're sending the message that food (especially low- or no-nutrient, sugary food) is linked to feeling good about yourself—encouraging emotional eating, in other words. For another thing, they're providing a whole new source of non-healthful foods that you can't control. Teachers in my son's school, sadly, do this a lot—and then wonder why there's a growing number of overweight children in the school district!

If this goes on in *your* children's school, approach the teacher or principal and voice your objections. If they object, saying that they need to provide incentives to get kids to perform, ask what's wrong with going back to giving out gold stars or stickers for good work. Or how about rewarding a child with a free period of arts and crafts. That's better for the mind *and* the body!

On the Physical Front

Parents can even insist on a tour of their children's school cafeteria to check out the conditions under which food is prepared for our kids. And if we don't like what we see, we can make our opinions known to the school and to the local school board. But be prepared for a challenge here. My experience working with school food-service providers has shown that, time and again, cafeteria workers resist offering healthier choices by claiming that the kids simply won't buy them. They've got the "bottom-line" mentality, where increasing school-lunch sales is more important than providing basic nutrition. However, when children are hungry and the food choices are appropriate, and there are no junk-food alternatives available—they'll eat what's offered *without a fuss*.

The same parental involvement is also necessary to restore physical activity to our children's school schedule. Daily activity—good, strenuous play, and sports—helps our kids develop in all sorts of ways, from improving general physical fitness and mental alertness to teaching teamwork and healthy competition. Just because our schools seem to have lost sight of this fact doesn't mean we have to sit back and accept the situation. After all, we pay for our schools through taxes or, in the case of private schools, through tuition and fees that have been skyrocketing in recent years. We need to make our voices heard!

Looking Ahead

As you can see, there are lots of ways in which our values, assumptions, and lifestyle choices can have an influence, for good or for ill, on our how our children think about food and fitness. And since the health of our children is, or should be, our first concern, we need to take the time to question our own attitudes—and the attitudes of our society—to see where we can improve things. It can sometimes appear too daunting a challenge—after all, we are living in a pretty high-stress world today, and sticking with the status quo may appear to be the easier way to go. But don't despair. As you read through the later chapters of this book, you'll learn lots of ways you can take charge of this fundamental part of your child's chances to adopt a healthy lifestyle!

THE MEDIA AND
ITS MESSAGE

3

*W*hen it comes to issues of health, safety, and nutrition, we're faced with a pretty big question: Just *who* is raising our children?! It seems as if the media is everywhere in our lives today, and especially everywhere in our *children's* lives. Through everything from music CDs to cable TV, from movies and videos to major sporting events, computer games, and Websites, major corporations are playing an ever-increasing role in what our children see, do, and listen to. They've even invaded our schools, as you'll recall from the previous chapter.

Why all this hyping to children? Simple economics! Every year, companies spend more than $2 billion advertising to kids—and you know it's not because they're *losing* money on the deal. In fact, in the November 2000 issue of *Entrepreneur* magazine, it was reported that the 12-to-19 year old age group spent about $94 billion of their own money on food, clothes, and accessories in 1998 alone! That's a market that no self-respecting greedy corporation can ignore!

PUMPING UP THE VOLUME

When you and I were kids, companies—and marketing firms —respected family values and the vulnerable naivete of youngsters. Sure we had Tony the Tiger and Ronald McDonald ads, but their impact was not nearly as tremendous as it is today. For one thing,

31

the sheer volume of advertising was less back then, and the advertising was clearly marked for what it was. Today, however, this has changed dramatically. Don't believe me? Try this simple experiment: next time your children are watching Saturday morning cartoons, take a break and watch with them. You'll be shocked to see just how many of the commercials feature high-sugar cereals and snacks. Even the advertisers seem to recognize that this is something they're "getting away with"—they're not so blatant with their advertising during the evening hours because they know that parent's are more likely to be watching, too. But when it comes to programming during Saturday mornings and the after-school hours of 3 to 5 pm, they're counting on us being too busy to notice!

As the networks discovered the vast revenues to be collected by selling advertising time, commercial breaks have expanded immensely: now the time devoted to actual programming is almost equal to the time spent on the commercials. And even within the shows themselves, corporate advertising is inescapable—thanks to the concept of "product placement." Once again, this is a relatively new phenomenon. If you catch re-runs on "nostalgia" channels like Nick-At-Night and TVLand, you'll be struck by the way these shows were careful to use generic packaging—no brand names allowed. When today's kids tune in to watch their favorite shows, however, they're getting a hefty dose of marketing as well. The logos and labels aren't just included in the scenes, they're prominently featured! If the TV Mom is making breakfast, you can bet that there's an open cupboard crammed full of Count Chocula or Cap'n Crunch cereal on display.

The problem is even more blatant in movies. Corporations make deals to get their products featured prominently in major motion pictures. The most extreme example, of course, is the hit Tom Hanks film, *Cast Away*—which was a full-length advertisement for Federal Express! But food manufacturers are no slouches in this regard either. Soft drinks are huge offenders in the product placement market—a recent example was the *Back to the Future* movie series, in which Pepsi was all over the place!

Every corporation is out for profit, and they've gotten so greedy that they've gone to extremes. There are *Harry Potter* tie-ins with fast-food restaurants and Coca Cola, and even the old "EZ-Bake Ovens" for kids come with McDonald's apple pie mix, while Play Doh comes with little Taco Bell and McDonald's stores!

Sometimes you've got to wonder if the executives of these companies have children of their own? The prevalence of this kind of thing has gone beyond advertising—and has become a form of brainwashing!

JUST WHAT ARE WE TEACHING OUR KIDS?

We live in a very hypocritical nation. Our lawmakers constantly talk about "better health care" and "better education opportunities" for our children—but with the same breath they deny the need to place controls on advertising. And no wonder—the same corporations that demand the right to saturation-advertising directed at children are making major campaign donations to these very same lawmakers during election years—and they've got some pretty powerful lobbyists in Washington who play a major role in picking and choosing which issues will get addressed. A case in point is Phillip Morris—best known as a cigarette manufacturer, but that's not their whole story. Along with their most famous cancer-causing product, they're also one of the major purveyors of junk food too! Here's just a partial list of their holdings:

Subsidiaries of Phillip Morris Company	
Breyers (ice cream and yogurt)	Louis Rich (cold cuts)
Cracker Barrel (cheese)	Minute Rice
Capri-Sun (sugar water)	Post cereals
Crystal Light (artificially sweetened water)	Oscar Meyer (cold cuts, hot dogs, Lunchables)
Shake N Bake (salt and sugar coating in a bag)	Philadelphia Cream Cheese (now offering "cream cheese snack bars" too)
Cool Whip (whipped topping)	Country Time (lemonade)
DiGiorno (pasta, pasta sauce, frozen pizza)	Taco Bell (fast-food, bottled salsa, taco mixes)
Good Seasons (salad dressings)	Stove Top (stuffing)

Subsidiaries of Phillip Morris Company, continued	
General Foods (cereals, crackers)	Tombstone (frozen pizza)
Jell-O (gelatin and puddings)	Tang (even more sugar water)
Kraft (cheese, macaroni and cheese mixes)	Velveeta (processed cheese stuff, macaroni and cheese mix)
Kool-Aid (more sugar water)	

These are clearly *NOT* your typical nutrient-dense food items, but mega-corporations like Phillip Morris routinely bring their political clout to bear in order to guarantee their own freedom to aggressively market these products to our kids!

The health and well-being of our children is obviously not a real priority—not when we actively encourage our food industry to push products that contain over 50 percent fat, tons of sugar, and more chemicals than actual 'real food.' And while we're on the subject—it's even more alarming to note that the stuff being advertised to kids is far less healthy than even the food that's advertised for adults! Take the example of a single—supposedly healthy—food: yogurt. One brand manufactures a product that features brightly colored sugar crystals—to give it more "kid appeal." Have you ever spilled a drop or two of that substance on your counter? It's nearly impossible to remove the stain! Can you imagine what it's doing to the stomach lining of your child?! Or how about the supposedly healthy "fruit-based" products— high-sugar, leathery "roll-ups" that are marketed to kids because they can be used to create temporary *tattoos* on the skin!! They are so far removed from *real* food that even the manufacturers don't dare try to pass them off as true fruit: they call it FROOT, instead.

BRIGHT COLORS, LOUD NOISE, AND ABOVE ALL, ACTION!

The junk-food industry has definitely taken notice of the huge market that our children represent—so they've made a point of educating themselves on how best to attract these young consumers (which is really how they see our kids). That long-running kid's show on public television, *Sesame Street*, provided the first real clues about how to grab and keep the attention of our nation's youngest consumers—it used bright colors, fast editing, and quirky, cartoonish characters to "sell" kids on learning their ABCs, and it worked! (Sadly, their innovative educational approach eventually took a turn for the commercial: now that it is corporately underwritten by AOL, it has lent its popular Elmo character to a blatant marketing ploy, showing Elmo with a dancing computer that sings the "You've Got Mail" jingle associated with the AOL e-mail service. And if you go to the Sesame Street Website, you'll spot a hyperlink to AOL at the very top of the list of corporate sponsors.)

Manufacturers of child-oriented products—including the food industry—were quick to pick up on the huge success of *Sesame Street.* They began employing market-research firms like Griffin Bacal, Inc., which produces the *Kidcurrents* newsletter dedicated to designing advertising strategies that specifically target children. The food industry quickly began to tailor its advertising specifically to young children, because they knew that by doing so they could influence two consumer groups for the price of one: they realized that not only do kids spend their own money, but they also have a lot of influence on what their *parents* will buy.

And what have they learned from all that marketing research? They've learned to make their commercials for kids more colorful, more dazzling, more exciting than the ones geared toward adults. They spend huge amounts of money coming up with catchy jingles that the kids will remember. (And we parents are not immune—how often have you caught yourself humming the jingle of a food commercial?) The corporations know that if they can catch a kid's attention, he or she will soon be *begging* Mom and Dad to buy their products!

McDonald's was one of the first companies to really catch on to this marketing strategy. Remember when *everybody* under the age of 18 was trying to sing the "two all-beef patties" jingle for the Big Mac? That was only the beginning! A survey of American children, published in Eric Schlosser's *Fast Food Nation: The Dark Side of the All-American Meal* (Houghton Mifflin Co. 2001), reported that 96 percent of them knew who Ronald McDonald was, and that the only character more popular than him was Santa Clause!

How did McDonald's do this? By targeting the kid's market directly. They introduced colorful, cartoon-like characters: Ronald McDonald, of course, but also the Cheese Burglar and talking French fries. They began offering specially packaged "kiddie meals" with tie-ins aimed at children's fascination with collecting: tiny toy figures or sets of drinking glasses and mugs featuring their trade-marked characters. And McDonald's' advertising strategy really paid off for the company—it grew from 1,000 restaurants in 1968 to 23,000 in 1998. The corporation opens 2,000 new restaurants every year! In 1970, Americans spent a whopping $6 billion on fast-food. In 1997, that market had grown to $100 billion, and in 2000, it topped $110 billion. Not bad, when you realize that the fast-food industry as a whole spends just $4 billion on advertising its products today!

The success of McDonald's was quickly copied by its competitors in the industry. Before long, all the other fast-food franchises had their own catchy jingles, special meal deals, and kid-friendly characters. And then came the biggest breakthrough of all—tie ins with kid-oriented movies! Soon we, as parents, were besieged with pleas for Happy Meals just so our kids could get one of the *Star Wars* or *Pokemon* action figures, just two of the most popular. And even if you wanted to avoid the junk food and just acquire the promo toy, you were stuck paying the full cost of the meal! As a result, according to Schlosser, the amount of money Americans spend today on fast-food is now actually more than we spend on movies, books, magazines, newspapers, videos and recorded music *COMBINED*!

BANG FOR THE BUCK?

Fast-food became popular because they offered a cheap way to get a hot meal. And, yes, it *is* cheaper to feed a family at most fast-food restaurants than at the more conventional, sit-down restaurants. But saving money by ordering food of limited nutritional value is not really saving, is it?

FROM CHILDHOOD TO TEEN YEARS

The kid's market isn't the only place where advertisers have identified easy profits. Teenagers are an equally attractive target: a few marketing dollars planted there can reap a huge harvest of profits. Why? Because teenagers have a great deal more discretionary control over how they spend their cash than their younger siblings do. And teenagers are very vulnerable to marketing—although they're more than willing to rebel against their parents, they're desperate to fit in with their peers. So if advertisers can convince the adolescent market that something is "cool," the pressure to conform can be very hard to resist.

Here again, advertisers have proven themselves to be more than willing to sacrifice responsibility for the sake of profits and, here again, our lawmakers are unable—or unwilling—to do anything about it. After all, how many decades did it take to get "Joe Camel" (the cigarette-smoking hipster cartoon) outlawed? And that was a cigarette-marketing campaign aimed directly at CHILDREN! Can we expect our legislators to work any more quickly on less obvious hazards to our children's health?

The Need to be "Cool"

As our children approach their teen years, they become more susceptible to marketing that's aimed directly at them. This is in part because they have greater control over their own spending money than their younger siblings. But there's another, more subtle factor at work as well. Adolescents are acutely conscious of their status. They feel like adults, and want to be treated that way. But at the same time, most of them are still discovering who it is they want to be—they haven't yet developed a strong sense of self. All they really know is that they want to fit in.

So as they enter their teen years, our children are actively looking for role models. Our celebrity-conscious society provides lots of people for our kids to emulate—some inspiring, some pretty dreadful—and we, as parents, have a tough fight on our hands to make sure that our own values get a fair hearing! It's hard to compete with a major sports hero or the current reigning rock star when you're trying to teach your kids about healthy living.

The idea of using celebrities as "product spokespersons" is hardly new—General Mills was an early leader in this, using the images of Olympic champions and other sports heroes on the front of their Wheaties breakfast cereal box. In the year 2000, gold medalists appeared on boxes of Frosted Flakes and Crispix, too. And today Kelloggs claims the honor of being the U.S. Olympic team's supplier through the year 2004 (as do McDonald's and Coca Cola).

Do you really think that, if given a choice, Olympians would choose Big Macs or Coke for their meals while they're training for competitions? It's true that companies like McDonald's have been corporate sponsors for the Olympics, and that they even made meals available for the participating teams. But the teams have a wide array of other foods as well—everything from grilled Tasmanian salmon to chicken with saffron rice! And keep in mind the difference in sheer energy level between competing sports participants and the average teenager—an athlete in training works off thousands of calories daily, so basically anything they eat is burned for fuel.

And sports figures aren't the only celebrities hired by food industry advertisers that want to attract the teen market. The soft-drink industry has long employed top pop stars to perform in elaborate videos—Michael Jackson and, more recently, Britney Spears being perhaps the most famous in this regard. And, of course, product placement in teen-oriented movies is a multi-million dollar business, a phenomenon that really took off during the 1980s and shows no sign of slowing. Meanwhile, the dieting industry is hiring major movie stars and even British royalty to tout their weight-loss programs.

Celebrities and Self-Image

Even more distressing, however, is how the food industry takes advantage of the insecurities of our teenagers, sometimes in very subtle ways. This is, after all, the time when children are acutely conscious of how they look. And the media is telling them that "skinny is in." On TV and in the movies, the happy and successful characters are all rail-thin, while the "dorky" kid—the "loser"—is always chubby, if not downright obese.

Look at the way characters are portrayed on TV. Slovenly types like Roseanne Barr and John Goodman (on the *Roseanne* show) are depicted as just a cut above trailer trash—not somebody that teen-agers or preteens want to emulate. On the other hand, the waif-like women on *Friends* are hugely popular, as are *Ally McBeal* and the heroine of the huge teen-hit, *Buffy the Vampire Slayer*. Meanwhile, the commercials that run through these programs push McDonald's and Burger King, Coke and Pepsi—how hypocritical can they *get!?* In this image conscious society, our vulnerable pre-teens and teenagers are very likely to internalize these attitudes about "attractiveness," and become highly critical of their own looks.

False Promises

Is it any wonder, then, that even while we're suffering a society-wide trend toward obesity, we're also seeing a sharp increase in adolescents suffering from eating disorders? And that trend is influenced in part by marketing practices and the media. The national obsession with thinness has led to more and more products being pushed on the public that have nothing to do with nutrition and everything to do with playing on our fears of fat.

Billions and billions of dollars are spent each year advertising fake foods—foods that promise to be fat-free, sugar-free, or "lite." Alongside of these questionable contributions to the nation's food cupboards are nutritional supplements and "herbal" or "energy" drinks and snacks. The idea is that you can buy your way to the ideal body, if you only can pick the right, ready-made products. The profits in this market are huge, so it's no wonder that advertisers are willing to spend their marketing dollars in an attempt to convince us that 'real' food is detrimental to our health.

And while we've been concentrating on television and the movies, the print media is equally involved. You don't need to look far for magazine articles and ads pertaining to weight loss and body image. They're everywhere! Even the supposed 'health'-oriented magazines contain monthly articles on the subject. Take a look at a few titles featured in the January 2002 issue of *Fitness*, a popular publication aimed at athletic, health-oriented individuals: "You <u>Can</u> Change Your Body" promises one, and "Eight Top Moves to Blast Fat Now" offers another (promising you that you'll get your "dream body" if you follow their advice). Is it possible to like yourself when print media is telling you not to?

And while we're being bombarded with media images that push the old (false) adage that "you can never be too thin," there are entrepreneurs out there just itching to jump in and make a quick buck off of our—and our vulnerable teenage daughters'—insecurities. Look at the weight loss industry: Over $35 billion dollars are spent on diet programs, pills, and potions that promise us a no-effort route to the perfect physique. But face it, if there really was a miracle cure available, we'd all be fit and healthy, and the weight-loss industry would be out of business! So do you think they *really* want us to succeed at weight loss and good health? Instead, the diet-industry is reaping huge profits, while obesity in America keeps growing every year!

MISPLACED MARKETING PRIORITIES

You never see commercials for fresh fruits and veggies, but you often see headlines touting the latest food contamination scare—pesticides, genetic manipulation of foodstuffs, and so on. It seems as if the media is going out of its way to drive us away from healthy eating. The only exception seems to be the recent ad campaigns promoting milk—but even that can be seen as the dairy companies' cynical manipulation of the fears of aging baby-boomers who are concerned about osteoporosis.

Instead, advertisers claim the "healthy eating" high ground but push less healthy, misleading—and even downright bad-for-you—products. For example, there are lines of frozen entrees that promote themselves as "Healthy Choice" or "Smart Ones" and imply that they're more healthful than their competition. But while there may be reduced sodium and less fat in these products, they're still misleading, because the portions are usually inadequate to satiate you, so you end up heading back to the kitchen for something more, just to satisfy your hunger.

And in many cases, the products live up to their claims of "low-fat" by replacing natural nutrients with chemicals—some of which can be pretty obnoxious if you think about them. For example, there's that fat replacement called Olestra, used in snack foods like potato chips. It's a chemical substance that looks and feels like fat when it's incorporated in food, but it was engineered to be completely indigestible by the human body—it passes right through without a bit of it being absorbed. The problem is that eating too many Olestra-laden potato chips can cause some pretty unpleasant side effects for many people. Check the label and you'll see a warning that the product can cause diarrhea and "anal leakage"! Mmmm-mmm, good, right? And notice that the "No Fat" claim appears in huge print on the front of the package, while the warning appears in teeny, tiny print on the back!

What's the point of all this? Simple. Manufacturers, and the marketers who push their products, have profits as their prime concern. As long as you can sell one more bag of snacks today, who cares what you're doing to the health of your consumers tomorrow? Even worse, if you can catch consumers while they're still young, you have a chance of building such strong brand loyalty that you can keep them for life—and they'll probably never even read those pesky small-print warnings on the back of your products.

FOOD LABELING PLOYS

While we're on the subject of food labels, there are a few things you should know. Most people think that the government has rules about truth in advertising. They tend to believe that if a company makes a claim about its product, it has to be true. Well, there really are laws about truth in advertising. For example, a product can not call itself "pork and beans" if there's mostly beans and only a little bit of pork—the first food item in the product name must be the item that forms the bulk of the product. But the loopholes are big enough to drive a truck through!

Taking Advantage of Trends

For example, look at how manufacturers abuse a simple word like "wheat." In the 1980s, Americans began rejecting white bread, heeding the health community's advice that we all needed more fiber in our diets. All of a sudden, "wheat bread" and "wheat crackers" became big sellers! Lots of companies rushed to put out products to take advantage of this new consumer craze—but often they did nothing more than toss a touch of wheat and a smaller touch of fiber into their original white-flour recipes. You've got to look closely at the labels—only those that use actual *whole* wheat give you the benefits you're looking for.

Then there was the "anti-cholesterol" craze. One prominent brand-name peanut butter rode that marketing bandwagon very effectively, touting their product as having ZERO cholesterol.

Hmmm. Since cholesterol is only found in animal products, and peanuts aren't animals, this particular brand was no different from any of its competitors—it never had cholesterol and neither did they! On the other hand, all peanut butter is high in fat—and that causes the body to make more of its *own* cholesterol (as you'll learn in Chapter 5).

And how about fruit juice drinks? Those should be pretty healthy, right? The problem is, many of these products are "made with," not "made of," real fruit juice. Check the labels and you'll often find that there's only 10 percent of real fruit juice (or less!). The rest is water with a little coloring and flavoring in to make it look and taste good. That means an 8-ounce serving gives you less than an ounce of real juice! Of course, this doesn't stop advertisers from claiming that their product is a "healthy" alternative—I remember one ad with a proud Mom watching as her kids root through the refrigeration, bypassing the carbonated drinks to reach for a brand-name juice product. The implication? They're presenting it as the healthy choice—but check the label and you'll see it's one of those 10-percent juice drinks!

And how about the way manufacturers jumped onto the "feathers and fins" craze a few years back. The media was touting the bad effects of saturated fat, which led to a crusade against red meats. Out of the woodwork came a whole slew of products that used to be made of beef but were now made with poultry—everything from turkey burgers to chicken hot dogs! These are supposed to be more healthful alternatives than their beef-based competition. It is true that fish, chicken, and turkey have less saturated fat than beef—if you serve the lean (white meat) portions and cut away all the fat and skin. But a look at the labels tells a different story—there you'll often find that the manufacturers have used dark meat and skin in the products.

Similarly, fish products enjoyed a huge upswing in popularity at about the same time. But when the product is breaded and fried, then smothered with a mayonnaise-based tartar sauce, the health benefits go right out the window!

Tailoring Their Pitch to Their Audience

And when the marketing people jump on a food-product bandwagon, they're likely to make—or imply—claims that have no scientific support whatsoever. Their only concern is to hit the "hot buttons" of the audience they're trying to reach. For example, the current craze is for "functional foods"—foods that are supposed to do more than just feed you. These foods represent the food industry's latest great marketing hope: concoctions of foods and herbal concoctions. And their prime audience is teens and young adults.

For example, there are chips made with St. Johns Wort, which is supposed to relieve your depression while you're enjoying your snack! Then there are iced teas with ginseng, and specialty foods and beverages designed to give you energy, sharpen your mind, improve your sex life, or protect your prostate. This is a manufacturer's and marketer's dream come true—if they can tightly define specialty niches, every person in the household will need a different kind of beverage, breakfast cereal, and snack food! Imagine your food bills—never mind the amount of storage space you'll need to stock all these things!

Sometimes this "niche" marketing can get a little strange. For example, consider how they market oatmeal. You'd think this would be the same no matter who they're selling it to, right? Think again. There are the "kid-oriented" ads, which stress the sugary flavors and simple preparation ("you can make your own!") of one line of oatmeal, while they're trying to hook Mom with a special "for women" brand that has extra calcium, taking advantage of the current buzz about the dangers of osteoporosis. Meanwhile, they're trying to market the old-fashioned, not-so-instant version as being particularly "hearth healthy." If you listen to the advertisers, you'd start to believe that you have to buy 3 entirely different kinds of oatmeal just to cover everybody's individual needs!

There Oughta Be a Law!

Certain claims are regulated—companies can't get away with slapping just *anything* on the label. For example, a specific health claim like "reduces the risk of heart disease" must be approved by the FDA. However, functional food claims are completely unregulated: claims like "designed to give you a burst of energy" are not subject to FDA scrutiny. The FDA relies on the manufacturer to be able to back up such claims with data, but no one ever really checks out either the data *or* the claim.

There are other ways food companies and their advertisers get around the rules. Changing the spelling of a key word, for example. To the public it seems like just a snappy advertising stunt, but it allows the manufacturers to imply that their product is something that it isn't. For example, there's precious little fruit in Froot Roll-Ups, but the manufacturer is breaking no rules by implying otherwise. Or stick the word "Lite" in the title—that can mean almost anything, but consumers are likely to assume that it is lower in fat and calories.

And sometimes advertisers just get a little tricky with the presentation of a product. You'll see high-sugar cereals featured in ads that claim they're "part of a healthy breakfast," and which show the table complete with orange juice, toast, and milk. The breakfast is only healthy when all the background food items are included! Meanwhile, the advertised cereal may be little more than a candy-coated starch in a breakfast bowl!

A big part of the problem is that much of the research that regulators rely on to check manufacturers' claims comes from biased studies. Manufacturers routinely employ their own experts to come up with research results that support company interests. For example, a Georgetown University research team recently published a study claiming that sugary soft drinks aren't as harmful as was once thought. The research group was in partnership with the Grocery Manufacturers of America and received grants from the Sugar Association—a clear case of conflict of interest.

Another suspicious study, published in the *Journal of the American Medical Association*, found that salt doesn't raise blood pressure. It was funded by the Campbell Institute for Research and Technology, part of the same firm that makes the high-sodium Campbell's line of canned soups. And then there's my all-time favorite: the study funded by the makers of Mars Bars that touts chocolate's benefit on heart health!

Have They No Shame?

It's really shameless how the corporations push truly junky foods on our kids. Everything is colored with dye, everything is excessively sweetened or salted, and everything is marketed as "fun, fun, fun"! All to get the kids to crave these products! And the tie-ins with toys just adds another layer of self-esteem damage: If Mom doesn't buy it for me, maybe she doesn't love me! It's hard to fight this kind of marketing manipulation, but that's what we have to do—because if our kids get caught up in this kind of thinking, they may end up paying for it for the rest of their lives.

The point is this: kids should be learning to eat because food is *good* for them. All these marketing messages confuse the issue—there are even toddler foods out there that push themselves as being kid-friendly: no sauce, so kids can play with their food without making a mess for Mom. Like we really need to encourage kids to play with their food! There are even products that suggest your children rub them on their bodies—they leave a wash-off tattoo behind! *None* of these serve a nutritional purpose, they only exist to boost the food manufacturer's profits.

IN THE STORE

Food manufacturers pay big bucks for the placement of their products. It pays to be displayed at the end of the aisles, near the check-out stands, and on the middle (eye level) shelves. Especially attractive are the shelves that are right about eye level for a child riding in the shopping cart—the manufacturers know that if they can catch a child's eye, the kids will bug his or her parents to buy it—especially if it contains a toy or other goodie featured prominently on the front of the box.

Other in-store ploys are specifically designed to get you to buy on impulse. That's why the bakeries are usually placed close to the check-out lines—hoping that you (or your kids) will be enticed by the smell of fresh-baked cookies. And that's why candy and other snacks are right there at the registers—they know that kids are likely to spot them and that parents will probably buy something just to avoid begging, whining, or even tantrums.

And even when it looks like you're getting a real deal, it's probably a much better deal for the manufacturer. Products that are "on special" at 3 for $5 might look like a bargain—but check the unit pricing and you'll probably find that the manufacturers are doing quite well for themselves. And buying three times more than you need of anything isn't a bargain—the more you have, the more you'll end up having to eat!

WHAT TO DO?

When it comes to kids, the problem is that they tend to believe what they see—they're not sophisticated enough to cut through the hype. Advertisers thrive on this, and present their products in ways that will hook a child's interest. They count on our kids to pressure Mom and Dad into buying products that we wouldn't normally consider bringing into the house.

The answer is to teach your children to be more savvy. Watch the television with them and point out how advertisers try to trick them. Explain that often the products look nothing like the TV version—and tell them that the idolized actor, athlete, or rock star is being paid a fortune to stand there with the product. But don't just preach at them—engage them in a real conversation, ask them what they think, get them started in the process of learning how to question what's presented instead of believing everything they see. You can make a game out of it. Kids *love* trying to catch somebody who is trying to trick them, so get your kids to try to spot the tricks: the meals that never look the same on the table as they do in the ads, or the great toy tie-in that's really just a boring hunk of plastic.

Keep a log of the amount of time your children spend in front of the TV. If it's upwards of 2 to 3 hours a day, they're spending *way* too much time being brainwashed by advertising. Encourage them to find other activities—reading, writing a story, doing crafts, or playing outside. And by all means, set guidelines for watching TV. It should come after more important activities, like doing homework, cleaning their rooms, walking the dog. Equally important, discourage television watching outside of the family's shared spaces—there's no reason for young children to have a television in their rooms. If they're locked away in their private space, you'll never be able to counteract the negative influences of programming and advertising, and you'll never have much shared family time!

THE MARCH OF TECHNOLOGY

4

$\mathcal{Y}$ou could say that technology is just another part of "life-style," and it's true that we discussed some aspects of technology and its effect on fitness and nutrition in Chapter 2. But technology —and by this I mean everything from the invention of the wheel to the development of genetically engineered foods—has had such a powerful influence on what we eat, when we eat, and how we eat, that it deserves a brief chapter of its own.

In this chapter we're going to take a close look at the specifics of how increasing technological development has sometimes worked against our developing a design for healthy living. We'll look at how technology has changed our very food supply, at how it has altered our general fitness level, and at how these changes have specifically impacted on our children. Finally, we'll revisit the issue of how technology has affected our interactions with one another, first raised in Chapter 2, to see how this has sometimes been detrimental to healthy living.

TECHNOLOGY AND OUR FOOD SUPPLY

Technology is not a late-20th century invention—technological innovation began when the first cave-person figured out how to make fire without waiting for lightning to strike a tree. And food and food production have been at the forefront of technological advance from the very start. Think about the "invention" of fire, for example. Sure it offered a means of lighting the caves, and it provided protection and warmth, but most of all it meant that food could be cooked—no longer did people have to eat everything raw.

There was good news and bad news with this, however. The good news was that foods that might have been inedible (too tough, too woody) could be made palatable by cooking. And it meant that foods could be kept longer, because cooking or smoking them kept them from spoiling so quickly. But often it meant that some nutrients were lost during the cooking process. The good news/bad news effect of technology on wellness has been with us ever since.

From Gathering to Farming

Another big technological leap was the shift from nomadic societies, which relied on gathering and hunting, to agriculture and raising livestock. The earliest societies really earned their daily calories—when out gathering the wild fruits, nuts, berries, and veggies, they covered huge amounts of territory, and hunting with your basic bow and arrow or spear took a lot of effort, too. Food processing was simple but labor intensive—lots of grinding and pounding was required to convert wild grains and nuts into something tasty to eat.

When people began farming, however, things changed dramatically. They began selectively breeding plants, choosing species that lent themselves to easy, predictable crops. At about the same time, they also started selectively breeding animals that were found useful for work or, more importantly, for food. This meant that people no longer had to cover huge territories to find enough to eat, and it meant that they could grow more than they needed—so some people didn't have to farm at all. Some people could work at other jobs, and there'd still be food for them to eat, as long as they had the money (or trade goods) with which to buy it.

Farming Becomes Big Business

The small farm's days were numbered when the Romans got into the act—they're the ones who invented the huge wheat farms you see all over the Mediterranean region, wherever Caesar made his conquests. But agriculture didn't really become a business for almost 1,500 years after that, and it wasn't until the middle of the twentieth century that full-scale, corporate agri-businesses—farms that combine agriculture with food-processing industries—really began to surface. The good news was that this development brought vast new opportunities to improve food production, so that more people could be fed by fewer farmers. The bad news, however, was that the control over the food supply was now almost exclusively in corporate hands. Why is this the bad news? Because, in the end, it is profitability, not quality, that counts within a corporation.

The Problem with Processing

A tomato is a tomato is a tomato. But the minute you start tinkering with that tomato, you've got a *product*! It can be ketchup, tomato paste, marinara sauce, or sun-dried. The profits for food producers are almost all found in the sale of these finished products —that's where the huge cost mark-ups can be built into the price of the product. So, if you're a corporation, you'd much rather get into the business of selling jars of marinara sauce than selling a plain old tomato—you can charge more for it.

In addition, you don't have to worry too much about the tomatoes you put into that jar of sauce. Nobody's going to buy a bruised or spoiled-looking vegetable or piece of fruit at the produce counter, but the food-processing company can pulp that shabby looking tomato up into a jar of sauce, add artificial coloring to make everything look tasty, add preservatives so it can sit on a shelf until it's sold, slap on a steep price—and everyone's happy, right?

In a nutshell, this is basically why the food industry would much rather tempt you into buying processed foods instead of the more wholesome fresh ingredients—the profit margin is so much better. But what's good for the industry comes at a higher cost to us, the consumers, than just the increased price of the food.

The Convenience Trade-off

The mid-1940s ushered in an age when the American consumers fell in love with the promise of convenience through technology, especially in the household. New appliances and processed foods were touted as being able to give the home-maker tons more free time and make cooking "a breeze." But although most of us probably wouldn't want to go back to baking all our own bread and spending hours cooking from scratch, these technological changes in our food supply haven't been an unmixed blessing.

Processing commonly strips much of the nutrient value from the ingredients, not to mention a lot of the flavor. To overcome these problems, the food manufacturers add enhancements to the product, fortifying them with some (but never *all*) of the nutrients that have been processed out of the original ingredients. And to build back some of the lost flavor (as well as to help preserve the product) they routinely add chemical flavorings and preservatives along with overwhelming amounts of sugar and salt—contributing to our excess intake of these items.

The result? In return for convenience, we get food at a much higher cost, with reduced food value and chemical additives that our bodies simply do not need. And more recent technological innovations have even reached down into our supply of raw materials —the basic veggies you buy at your local supermarket. For easier shipping, genetic researchers have come up with, of all things, square tomatoes—they're easier to pack up in crates. And while nothing can compare with the taste of real, farm-grown fruits and veggies, researchers are perfectly willing to come up with bland and tasteless produce, as long as it's gorgeous looking—because good-looking produce is easier to sell than its tastier, but less attractive, competition.

A Hopeful Shift

There is a small but growing movement that is beginning to challenge the trend toward highly processed and genetically manipulated foods in our supermarkets. Small local farms are gaining popularity in some areas, and nearly every supermarket now boasts a section devoted to "organically grown" produce and meats. Unfortunately, these products are often very pricey, and there's no standard definition of "organic," so you can't always be sure that you're getting pesticide- and preservative-free products, especially if you're buying them in a big name store or a national supermarket chain.

Your best bet? For fruits and veggies, it's a good idea to look for products that are grown locally and buy them in season. Most communities have farmers' markets or even roadside produce stands where you can be sure you're buying food that's at least been fresh-picked. Locally-grown foods are also usually less expensive than the "organic" foods in your supermarket, because local farmers don't have to build in extra costs to cover long-distance shipping fees.

TECHNOLOGY AND THE DECLINE IN FITNESS

Technology has had an equally dramatic impact on the general fitness levels in our country—and especially in our children. We've already mentioned (and it will come up again, for sure) the huge amount of time our children spend parked in front of the television—and with the spread of computers into almost every household, when kids aren't in front of the TV it seems they're playing computer games or hooked up to the Internet. But this is only the most recent example of how technology has contributed to the decline in our level of fitness.

Hitchin' a Ride

From the earliest times, humans have spent a great deal of energy trying to find ways to spend *less* energy. The invention of the wheel was just one of the first in a long line of labor-saving devices that led to the creation of everything from automobiles and airplanes to electricity and elevators. And each invention made it a little bit easier to cut back on the exercise we would otherwise have gotten. The most dramatic difference can be seen in our most basic activity—walking.

How often do you catch yourself hopping into the car to drive to the corner store? Or to bring your kids to a nearby friend's house to play? Not so long ago, those destinations were considered to be "in walking distance." But with 2- and 3-car households, it just seems easier to drive than to walk.

And our modern communities often work against us, as well. In the suburbs, developers ignored our nearby "downtown" areas in favor of malls, usually located on the far edges of the residential districts—and built our supermarkets out there, too. Big department store chains like Target took this a step further, adding food aisles alongside the housewares and clothing sections, offering one-stop shopping convenience.

Meanwhile, many people feel that our neighborhoods and streets are more dangerous these days—they just feel *safer* in a car than they do walking. It seems like we don't go *anywhere* on foot anymore, unless we make a conscious effort—jogging, for example, or working out on a treadmill. When we walk these days, it seems like most of the time we're walking to nowhere!

And, actually, these days we're just getting plain lazy. How many times have you found yourself circling the parking lot, trying to find the empty parking spot that's closest to the door? If we'd just park out in the "boonies" of the lot, we'd have a nice, manageable walk to the store, and we wouldn't have to spend so much time walking to nowhere on the treadmill!

Redefining Playtime

The change for our kids has been especially dramatic. Safety concerns have made us less comfortable (or even downright fearful) about letting them "run loose" outside, so they have less opportunity to get involved in the active games and sports that were common in the past. Activity has become something to be scheduled—sign the kids up for the local soccer team or Little League. But there aren't enough teams for every kid, and let's face it—lots of parents don't have the time or the resources to get their children involved.

At home, play options have also become limited. Active games like *Tag, Kickball,* or *Hide and Seek* require multiple players—not easy to come by if few kids live in your neighborhood. So games like *Twister*—which involves a fair amount of activity but requires a bunch of kids to make it fun—have been replaced by more solitary pursuits. Besides, how can an old-fashioned game like that compete with the glitzy excitement of video games?

And don't fool yourself with the idea that kids are probably making up for all this lost exercise while they're in school. School exercise programs have been dramatically cut back in most places —just over one-third of our elementary and middle schools offer daily physical activity to all the children, while most offer it only once or twice per week! And as our schools face their own security concerns, fewer and fewer offer unstructured, active play outdoors during recess.

According to the Surgeon General's report on physical activity and health, activity levels decrease as kids get older, and really drop off as kids enter adolescence. Nearly half of youngsters age 12 to 21 are not vigorously active, 25 percent engage in no vigorous activity, and a full 14 percent report no recent activity, even at light levels. Girls are more likely to be inactive than boys, especially once puberty hits. But the gender gap occurs even with younger kids—it seems that parents are more likely to let boys go out and play on their own!

What's the result? Our kids are getting much less physical activity each day than ever before. They're driven everywhere and participate in formal sports rather than getting their own games together. Conscientious parents try to compensate by signing their kids up for scheduled playtime—I've personally enrolled my son in judo, hockey, and (depending on the season) soccer or baseball, just to make sure he gets in enough vigorous exercise. I don't want him to end up filling his playtime with activities that require almost no movement at all, except for his mouse-clicking finger!

Is your child at risk? Pick a day when you've got time to spare and keep track of how much time your children spend in *real* active movement. If your family is like most, you'll be shocked to see how much time is spent without exercise at all.

RELATIONSHIPS IN THE AGE OF TECHNOLOGY

Increased technology has also had a negative impact on human—especially family—relationships, with dire consequences for our kids' overall fitness. This is a tricky problem to understand, but it *is* important!

Where Have all the Playmates Gone

First of all, our children have far fewer opportunities for active play. You've already seen how changes in our communities have basically extinguished the old neighborhood full of kids who could feel safe just roaming free. Games just aren't as much fun when there's only one or two kids around. It's much easier to bide time watching a favorite video, surfing the Internet or playing with an X-Box.

Some parents have tried to overcome this lack of social play by setting up "play-dates" for their kids, scheduling times when one adult is free to supervise the children. Too often, however, even these social opportunities end up being spent in low- or no-activity entertainment. And, of course, once kids reach a certain age, they're likely to resist such adult-organized events.

Home Alone and Lonely

In this age of latchkey kids and two-income households, we've come to rely on television, video games, and the Internet as a baby-sitter. This means that a lot of our children spend a great deal of "alone-time." This has a subtle effect on their well-being that many parents don't really see.

For kids, being alone can mean being lonely, and with that loneliness can come depression. By definition, depression is linked to lethargy, and a depressed person—even a child—can find it very difficult to get active. Even worse, it's easy to turn to food as a way to comfort yourself when you're depressed—emotional eating, which is not a good habit to let your kids get into.

The problem isn't "just a phase" that kids grow out of, unfortunately. Depressed and lethargic kids too often turn into depressed, lethargic, and unproductive adults. And when you add in the influences of the media—negative messages in TV programs and movies, violent video games, and so on—no wonder lots of kids have a hard time developing a healthy moral sense.

The problem—beyond the fact that none of us want our children to feel depressed—is that the less activity a child has, the more the lethargy can intensify and the deeper the depression can become. As time goes on, it becomes harder and harder to motivate such a child to do much of anything except retreat into favorite pastimes—which, too often, are passive pursuits like watching TV or escaping into a video game.

Communications Breakdown

As our kids become increasingly immersed in technology, they spend less time directly relating to the people around them. The universe of a video game is attractive to kids because they feel as if they're in control of something pretty big and exciting. And surfing the Internet, too, gives a sense of control—a shy, nerdy kid can be anybody he or she wants to be in a chat room.

The problem here is that these outlets are very seductive to our kids. Nobody in the chat room knows that little Suzie or little Joey is only 8 or is having trouble with their homework. Mom and Dad—and brother and sister—on the other hand, know these things all too well. So little Joey and little Suzie often prefer spending time with their virtual friends, who never remind them of their downfalls and never make fun of them, as the real people in their lives sometimes do.

This often means that the communication between and among family members suffers. Without sufficient communication, it becomes virtually impossible to teach your family values and your morals to your children. Suddenly, the advice or attitudes of an animated cartoon character, or a nameless, faceless, virtual buddy carries more weight than yours does. (And in this age of Internet predators, this can get *really* scary!)

Competing Messages

Most difficult of all, however, is the fact that parents in this high-tech, media-dominated age have to compete with so many overwhelmingly "loud" messages. The sad thing is many are in direct opposition to what we're trying so hard to teach our kids. You may work very hard to explain why good nutrition is important, but then up pops a commercial for a "must-have" collectible —available with the purchase of a Happy Meal! Or a new-on-video movie ("guaranteeing *hours* of happy viewing") that the kids watch over and over again rather than going outside to play. Or a Froot Roll-up they can wear as a tattoo.

Finally, there's the view of the world that these high-tech playmates offer—a world where skinny or buff is everything, and where normal-bodied people are presented as losers (remember *Roseanne?*). Kids are very sensitive about "fitting in," and the general message presented in the glossy world of tech can easily make them feel personally inadequate. The damaging effect of such low self-esteem is often realized in behavior that is damaging to our kids' health—depression, anxiety, eating disorders, and other self-destructive behaviors.

MARCHING TO A NEW BEAT

In the last few chapters we've explored the many factors that work against our children's health and fitness. By now it may seem almost impossible to overcome all of these obstacles working against us—but don't give up hope! There really are *lots* of ways you can take back control of the situation and turn it around. With a solid understanding of the basic facts of fitness and nutrition, especially for kids, and a solid plan—a Design for Healthy Lifestyles—you'll have all the tools you need to introduce your children to the rewards of food, fun, n' fitness!

Part Two

Ages and Stages

5

FOOD
FUNDAMENTALS

The key to well-balanced nutrition is variety. You want to plan meals that include a wide range of foods, because no one food or food group contains every nutrient your body needs.

In this chapter, you'll learn about the different types of foods you eat, and how they help you meet your nutritional needs. We'll start with a look at the way that foods—and the nutrients they contain—are classified and categorized, and then we'll take an in-depth look at some of the most important elements of a sound, healthy diet. After that, we'll look at a few "special" nutrients that are vital to a child's growth, health, and well being, but which aren't as easily obtained as some of the more abundant nutrients. Sometimes you have to make an extra effort to ensure that your child gets an adequate supply of these "special" nutrients. But isn't it worth it?

AN INTRODUCTION TO
FOOD CATEGORIES

Over the years, nutrition experts have come up with many different ways to categorize and classify our food requirements. Although the individual techniques differ, the underlying principles are the same. Perhaps the most familiar of all these techniques is the Food Guide Pyramid, developed by the U.S. Department of Agriculture (USDA).

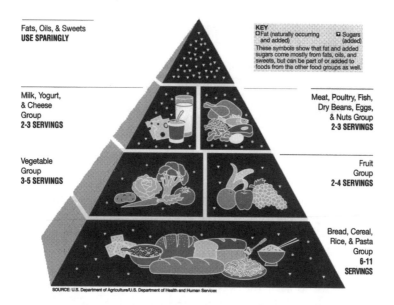

Food Guide Pyramid

A Guide to Daily Food Choices

Fats, Oils, & Sweets
USE SPARINGLY

KEY
☐ Fat (naturally occurring   ▨ Sugars
  and added)   (added)
These symbols show that fat and added
sugars come mostly from fats, oils, and
sweets, but can be part of or added to
foods from the other food groups as well.

Milk, Yogurt,
& Cheese
Group
2-3 SERVINGS

Meat, Poultry, Fish,
Dry Beans, Eggs,
& Nuts Group
2-3 SERVINGS

Vegetable
Group
3-5 SERVINGS

Fruit
Group
2-4 SERVINGS

Bread, Cereal,
Rice, & Pasta
Group
**6-11
SERVINGS**

SOURCE: U.S. Department of Agriculture/U.S. Department of Health and Human Services

Use the Food Guide Pyramid to help you eat better every day. . .the Dietary Guidelines way. Start with plenty of Breads, Cereals, Rice, and Pasta; Vegetables; and Fruits. Add two to three servings from the Milk group and two to three servings from the Meat group.

Each of these food groups provides some, but not all, of the nutrients you need. No one food group is more important than another — for good health you need them all. Go easy on fats, oils, and sweets, the foods in the small tip of the Pyramid.

To order a copy of "The Food Guide Pyramid" booklet, send a $1.00 check or money order made out to the Superintendent of Documents to: Consumer Information Center, Department 159-Y, Pueblo, Colorado 81009.

U.S. Department of Agriculture, Human Nutrition Information Service, August 1992, Leaflet No. 572

Source: USDA

The USDA Food Guide Pyramid is a visual representation of our daily food needs, displayed as a triangle in the approximate proportions necessary for adequate nutrition. Foods are broken down into six categories, with the cereals and grains taking up the biggest space at the bottom. Fruits and vegetables come next, in about equal proportions, followed by somewhat smaller servings of dairy on one side and meats, beans, eggs, and nuts on the other. At the very top are fats, oils, and sweets. But to understand what the pyramid is really telling us about proper nutrition, we have to understand how the categories were established. That means under- standing something called the "Dietary Guidelines."

FROM RDA TO RDI TO DIETARY GUIDELINES

For many years, the Recommended Dietary Allowances (RDAs) were the gold standard for determining whether or not you were getting enough of a range of necessary nutrients. Extrapolated by the USDA from solid scientific research, the RDAs listed the specific amounts of the essential nutrients we need, adjusting these amounts to reflect the specific needs of particular age groups and the different nutritional needs of males and females. For a long time, RDAs were the only nutritional guide used by health and nutrition professionals, but they suffered from some real limitations —specifically, they failed to take into account individual variations in height, weight, and activity level.

To address these pitfalls, a new nutritional standard has been developed. It's known as the Recommended Dietary Intake, or RDI. Like the RDAs, the RDIs give specific amounts of the essential nutrients for various age and gender categories, but they incorporate other information as well, and can therefore be applied to a broader population than the RDAs.

The RDI system still suffers from one problem, however. Like its predecessor, it is too "mathematical" and too cumbersome for most non-professionals to use effectively. To address this problem, the Dietary Guidelines and the Food Guide Pyramid are used to translate the RDIs into a format that most people can easily understand.

The Dietary Guidelines provide information and suggestions for the average consumer that can help us to make sound nutritional choices. In addition, it incorporates related information on fitness and activity. To keep the guidelines up-to-date, the USDA and the Department of Health and Human Services revise them periodically. Here's what the Guidelines for the year 2000 look like (you can view them for yourself on the Internet, at www.nal.usda.gov/fnic/dga/rda/pdf):

2000 Dietary Guidelines = ABC

Aim for Fitness
— Aim for a healthy weight
— Be physically active each day

Build a Healthy Base
— Let the pyramid guide your food choices
— Eat a variety of grains, especially whole grains
— Eat a variety of fruits and vegetables daily
— Keep foods safe to eat

Choose sensibly
— Choose a diet low in saturated fat and cholesterol and moderate in total fat
— Choose beverages and foods to moderate your intake of sugars
— Choose and prepare foods with less salt
— If you drink alcoholic beverages, do so in moderation

Now let's look at each of these guidelines, one at a time:

"Aim for Fitness" means establishing a *realistic* weight for your lifestyle—one you can maintain without eating like a bird or running marathons every day. At the same time, the guidelines call for reasonable activity—walking when you can, taking stairs instead of elevators, and so on.

"Build a Healthy Base" means paying attention to food choices and making sure that your daily diet includes appropriate amounts from each of the basic food groups in the Food Guide Pyramid. It also means striving for variety within the fruit and grain categories, because if you eat the same foods day in and day out, you may be missing out on important nutrients. It reminds you that whole grains, fresh fruits, and veggies are an important part of a healthy daily diet. And it means paying attention to the quality and safety of the food you prepare and eat. Many fruits and vegetables are coated with pesticides, so make sure they're washed thoroughly before cooking. Check the expiration dates on perishables. Thoroughly cook foods, especially meats and poultry, to kill bacteria. And wash all preparation surfaces and implements—as well as your hands—after you're done.

Finally, "Choose Sensibly" means cutting back on excess. For example, you can cut back on extra fat by reducing the amount of butter you use on your baked potato—or replace it entirely with one of the low-fat or fat-free substitutes that are available these days. You can cut back on cholesterol by reducing the amount of animal-derived foods you eat, since cholesterol is only found in animal products. And you can moderate your sugar intake by opting for milk instead of soft drinks, or choosing a piece of fruit instead of sugary snacks. (Did you know that even chocolate has less sugar and more nutrients than an equal number of calories in the form of jelly beans or froot roll-ups?) And when it comes to cutting back on salt, try garlic, pepper, and other spices to add flavor, instead of reaching for the salt shaker.

CLIMBING THE PYRAMID

The Dietary Guidelines for Americans are helpful, but they can't stand alone—you need to refer to the Food Guide Pyramid to get more specific advice about how much of each food type you should eat each day. The Food Guide Pyramid classifies food as: 1) milk and dairy products; 2) meat and meat alternatives; 3) fruits and veggies; 4) bread, cereals, and grains; 5) fats and oils; and 6) "others"—basically sugars. The Pyramid makes the following general recommendations regarding servings per day for each food class, and tells you how to calculate the size of a single serving:

Daily Amount	Serving Size
6 to 12 servings from bread	1 slice bread, 1/2 c noodles, 1/3 c rice/beans
3 to 5 servings meat	2 oz meat, fish, poultry, and meat alternatives; 2 Tbsp peanut or nut butter; 1 egg; 1/2 c legumes
3 to 4 servings dairy	8 oz milk or yogurt, 1 oz cheese, ½ c cottage cheese
3 to 5 servings veggies	1/2 c cooked, 1 c raw
2 to 3 servings fruit	1 medium fruit, 1 c melon or berries, ½ c juice
Fat as needed for calories	<3 tsp for under 5; <3 Tbsp for over 5

Keep in mind that the Food Guide Pyramid is not without its faults. For one, it doesn't place enough emphasis on the benefit of whole grains over refined flour products. Nor does it encourage high fiber foods and non-animal protein alternatives. And last but not least, the suggested serving sizes aren't exact. A person's actual intake depends on age, gender, activity level, and so on.

What I find shocking is that, based on the USDA estimates, only one percent of children aged 2 to 19 actually meet all the guidelines specified by the food guide pyramid!

KNOWING YOUR NUTRIENTS

It's all well and good to know the kinds of food you should be eating, but to really understand about nutrition, you need to know *why* you should be eating them. That means understanding the nutrients they contain and what those nutrients do for you. Nutrition experts spend years learning all about these things, getting into the nitty-gritty of how each nutrient breaks down in the body and so on, but you don't have to go that far. Instead, concentrate on learning *the basics*—which nutrients are important and why—so that you can better understand the importance of getting the right amounts of nutrients into your meals every day.

And just what are these important nutrients? Science has identified 6 categories of basic, necessary nutrients that the body needs to grow and maintain itself. These are:

Water

Protein

Carbohydrates

Fats

Vitamins

Minerals

These nutrients are the fuel and building blocks you need to keep healthy. They're especially important during childhood, when the body is growing and developing. Let's take a closer look at each one.

Water

Believe it or not, water is your body's most essential nutrient. Water does not provide calories or energy, but without it, none of us could survive. Depending on your age, water makes up 50 to 75 percent of your body weight—the younger the child, the greater the percentage of water in overall body weight: an infant is 75 percent water.

Water fulfills a number of important functions in the body. As the main component of blood, it provides the medium through which oxygen and all the other nutrients are transported to the cells of your body. It also helps to regulate body temperature and acts as a shock absorber, providing a protective cushion to protect major body tissues and organs, like the spinal cord and brain. It does other things as well, such as flushing your system of waste products through urine and keeping your body's electrolytes (sodium, potassium, and chloride) in balance. These electrolytes— minerals with an electrical charge—keep your body's fluids at the proper levels and help your muscles and nervous system to function properly.

Water allows your sense organs to function, too. For example, you hear sounds because of waves that are transmitted through a water-based fluid in the inner ear, and the fluid in your eyes permits light to be reflected, enabling you to see. Even your senses of smell and taste rely on water, which dissolves your food and releases their taste and aroma.

Because fluids (preferably water) play such an important role in maintaining a healthy body, it's important to make sure that we all get enough. As with all nutrients, the amount required varies according to age, gender, activity levels, and even environmental factors, such as exposure to heat. What's important to keep in mind is that if you don't get enough fluid, dehydration can occur very quickly. This is especially true for youngsters.

We get a lot of our water directly from the liquids we drink, but not all liquids are created equal. In fact, some liquids actually deplete us of water. Coffee, tea, and alcohol are actually *dehydrating*! They influence the hormones that regulate fluid balance, triggering your system to make more urine. And many soft drinks ultimately remove more fluid than they provide. This is because they contain salt and sugar, large molecules that must be diluted in the blood stream. As a result, they actually pull fluid from the cells during digestion, and the water is then flushed out of your system through urine.

Protein

Protein is another one of our most essential nutrients. It plays a part in a number of vital, body-building functions, and is especially important during childhood—a period of rapid growth. You see, the muscle tissue in our bodies is made up of protein; in fact, every organ in our bodies is made up of this essential nutrient.

Protein as muscle and other body tissues plays a big role in regulating the body's metabolism. How does this work? It is your muscle tissue that burns up the calories (energy) you consume in your food—a process known as metabolism. The more muscle you have, the higher your metabolism will be, and as a result, the more calories you will burn.

In addition to providing the building blocks for creating muscle, protein carries nutrients throughout the body, "hand-delivering" them to areas in need. It also helps assure there is enough blood circulating throughout the body and helps to strengthen the immune system, fighting infection and disease. It's necessary for making and regulating the hormones that control blood pressure and heart rate and is involved in growth and maturation. And, as enzymes, proteins create the signals that enable your cells to do their work—from contracting the muscles of the heart to sending electrical signals to your brain.

Protein is made up of amino acids, of which there are 20 in all. Your body can make a little more than half of these on its own. However, nine of them must be obtained through the food you eat. The ones your body makes on its own are, somewhat misleadingly, called *non-essential amino acids*, whereas the ones you can only get from the food you eat are called *essential* amino acids. But don't let the names fool you: all of them are equally important in order for your body to make protein.

Protein is found in foods derived from both animals and plants. Protein from animal products—beef, chicken, fish, lamb, veal, pork, and dairy products—is more readily digestible and therefore of a higher quality than that from plants. Plant-based protein is also good for you, but plant protein is only about 85 percent digestible, so you have to eat larger servings of vegetables, grains, or legumes to get the same amount of protein as you would get in a single serving of meat or dairy. Also, animal-based proteins contain all of the essential amino acids in a single source, whereas plant-based protein generally contains only some of them.

This is not to say that plant proteins aren't good for you—in fact, they have some benefits over animal protein, such as no cholesterol, much less fat, and rarely any saturated fat. They're also higher in fiber. And one of the meat alternatives—soy—is linked to a reduced risk of certain cancers.

Still, vegetarians must pay attention to "complementary proteins"—combining plant-protein sources to ensure that they're getting all the amino acids that their bodies need. For example, grain contains some of the essential amino acids, whereas legumes contain the others. Thus, a vegetarian will choose a dish made with both, like beans and rice or a bowl of minestrone soup. Nutritionists used to think that you had to combine these complementary proteins in the same meal, but more recent research indicates that its okay to eat them separately, as long as you get both protein sources within the same 24-hour period. But no matter where it comes from, protein has 4 calories per gram.

Carbohydrates

Carbohydrates are pretty easy to understand. Their main function is to provide the body with enough energy to get through the day—like putting gas in your car. The fuel we get from carbohydrates is a form of sugar, called glucose. The energy units contained in that glucose are what we call *calories.*

Almost everything we eat is converted to glucose for energy. However, your body usually doesn't need to use all the energy as soon as it is consumed. Rather than waste all that energy, your body converts it to fat or glycogen (which is the storage form of glucose), so that it can be stored for later use.

Simple or complex? There are two types of carbohydrates—simple and complex—distinguished by their physical structures. Simple carbohydrates are the sugars, which are made up of short chains of carbon, hydrogen, and oxygen atoms. Complex carbohydrates are called starches. These, too, are made up of carbon, hydrogen, and oxygen, but these elements are put together in longer, branched chains. The structural differences between sugars and starches make a difference in how your body handles them. Simple carbohydrates are more easily digested than their more complex, starchy counterparts, so they're a quick source of energy and they're rapidly metabolized.

The complex carbohydrates, on the other hand, are not only a great source of readily available energy, they are an excellent source of the B (or energy) vitamins, trace minerals, and much, needed dietary fiber. As such, they should form the major part of everyone's daily food intake. The best sources of complex carbohydrates include whole grain breads, cereals, brown rice, quinoa, amaranth, barley, millet, bulgur, and buckwheat, as well as legumes (beans) and vegetables. Whole fruits are a little special. The fructose in them is a simple carbohydrate, but the whole fruit contains fiber that helps slow its absorption. That's why eating whole fruit is better than just drinking the juice.

But regardless of whether the carbohydrates you eat are simple or complex, in the end they are all converted to glucose. Once glucose is formed, it can enter the blood and be used as energy the very minute it is produced, or it may be converted to glycogen or fat and then stored in the body for later use. If it is converted to glycogen, it will be stored in the liver or in muscle tissue. If it is converted to fat, it is stored in the body's adipose or fat tissue. If you really pig out on simple sugars—say, pounding down a lot of jelly beans or gummi bears in a single sitting—your body will be flooded with so much unneeded glucose that it will simply pass some of it through your system without processing it, and it will be excreted in the urine.

If you're old enough to read this, you've probably heard that carbohydrates—like bread and pasta—are fattening. Not so. Sure, they can be converted to fat for storage, but the problem is not in the carbohydrates, but rather in the *amount* of carbohydrates you consume. The problem with carbohydrates—and really with *all* the food groups—is portion size. We typically serve complex carbohydrates like pasta, rice, and beans in large quantities, and then add high calorie fats like butter or other sauces to them as well! Too much of *anything*, even a "good for you" food, is "fattening."

Fiber facts. Complex carbohydrates are the foods which provide bulk and fiber to the diet. Fiber makes you feel full faster than protein does, and with fewer calories. But not all complex carbohydrates are created equal. Recent research indicates the best complex carbohydrates are the least processed. In simple terms, whole-wheat bread is better than processed white bread; brown or long-grain rice is better than refined white rice; and bulgur, quinoa, and millet are better than noodles. Why? Much of the mineral and fiber content is stripped from grains when they are processed or refined. Manufacturers try to fix this by "enriching" their products—sort of like adding a vitamin pill to the flour—but they can't completely restore all the important parts of the grain that processing strips away.

So what's so important about fiber? Fiber is the part of any plant that cannot be digested by the body—when you eat it, you can't break it down into a usable nutrient. It provides the bulk that is necessary to keep your bowel function "regular," which helps your body to eliminate the waste by-products left after food is digested. Fiber also helps to slow down the absorption of food in the digestive tract. This helps regulate the rate by which you produce blood sugar (glucose). It also helps to produce a feeling of fullness, helping to keep you satiated longer.

Soluble and insoluble. There are 2 types of fiber: soluble and insoluble. Soluble fiber expands by absorbing water as it passes through your intestinal tract, forming a gelatin-like substance, whereas insoluble fiber passes through your system without any appreciable change. Both types, being bulky, help make you feel full after eating, and both help clear your intestinal tract of waste.

Soluble fiber offers other health benefits, too. For example, soluble fiber has been proven to improve heart health. It does this by transporting cholesterol to the liver, where the cholesterol is converted to bile acids and then excreted from the body. Oat bran, legumes, and the pectin in fruits and vegetables are all good sources of soluble fibers. Another source, previously used mainly in laxatives but recently endorsed for use in bran cereals by the FDA, is psyllium, which comes from a plant grown in India.

Insoluble fiber also has some health benefits beyond just keeping us "regular." It is believed to help prevent colon cancer because it reduces the amount of time it takes for digested food to pass through our intestines and bowel. Wheat bran, the cellulose in vegetables (such as the 'threads' in celery), and fruit are good sources of insoluble fiber.

The typical American consumes too little fiber. The American Dietetic Association recommends a daily fiber intake of 15 to 40 grams a day for adults, of which 5 to 10 grams should be soluble. The average daily consumption, however, is only 12 to 15 grams of total fiber a day, and only 3 to 4 grams of this is soluble fiber. Why are we getting so little fiber in our diets? Mainly because we don't eat enough fruits, vegetables, and whole grains.

Given how important fiber is to a healthy diet, it's a good idea to make sure you—and your kids—are getting enough. The recommendation for children is 5 grams plus 1 gram for every year they are old. So an 8 year old should strive for 13 grams (5 plus 8) per day. But be careful when you start increasing your fiber intake. Fiber is "bulking"—it can cause digestive discomfort if you increase your intake too quickly, and you must remember to increase your fluid intake at the same time as you increase your consumption of fiber.

Fat

I am sure everyone has heard all of the bad-mouthing going on about dietary fat. Fat has been accused of causing everything from obesity to heart disease to cancer. Well, if you tend to eat a very high-fat diet, most of this is true. But in moderation, fat is actually a *good* thing. You need it in order to process some of the vitamins your body needs. Vitamins A, D, E, and K are all "fat soluble," which means they can't be used by your body unless they are dissolved in fat.

Fat also acts as insulation, protecting the body from extreme temperatures. And it provides a protective cushion for your internal organs. In addition, fat, like fiber, helps slow the absorption of food in the digestive tract, which helps to produce a more stable energy level. And because fat contains more than twice as many calories per gram as protein or carbohydrates (9 calories for fat, 4 each for protein and carbohydrates) and takes about 6 hours to digest, you end up feeling more satisfied after a meal, for a longer period of time.

Variations on the fat theme. Fat comes in two varieties: saturated and unsaturated. Each type is distinguished by its chemical structure, but we don't need to go into a deep scientific lecture to understand the differences between them. Saturated fats are solid at room temperature, and they are blamed for clogging up our arteries. This makes sense when you consider that a person's body temperature is pretty close to "room temperature"—so saturated fats in your system are likely to solidify in your blood vessels. Saturated fat is found mainly in animal and dairy based foods—beef, pork, chicken, butter, eggs, and cheese. However, coconut and palm oils are also saturated fats.

There are two types of unsaturated fats: monounsaturated and polyunsaturated. The difference between the two is in the way the fat molecules are organized, but both usually remain in liquid form at room temperature, so they're not likely to solidify in your veins and arteries like saturated fats do. Polyunsaturated fats include corn and sesame seed oils, while monounsaturated fats include olive, safflower, canola, and peanut oils.

A subdivision of the polyunsaturated fats are the "omega's": the Omega-3 and Omega-6 fatty acids, both of which are considered to be important in the healthy development and functioning of the body. Omega-3s are found in fish like salmon, as well as canola, flaxseed, and walnut oils. Omega-6s are found in vegetable oils like corn and safflower. Like the monounsaturated fats, the omegas do not seem to increase blood cholesterol or blood fat (lipid) levels. It seems that they help to reduce the "stickiness" of platelets in the blood, which in turn helps prevent the build-up of plaque along artery walls.

The monounsaturated fats are now being touted as the new "good guys" of nutrition, capable of helping to lower cholesterol and prevent heart disease. If you must use a fat when preparing your food, this is the ideal choice. But while there are great health benefits associated with monounsaturated fats and with the omegas, keep in mind that, any type of fat, whether it be butter, margarine or olive oil, has 100 calories per tablespoon. That's not a heaping tablespoon either.

The cholesterol conundrum. Cholesterol has always been a concern of nutritionists, because of its potential for causing serious health problems. High cholesterol can cause a condition called atherosclerosis, commonly known as "hardening of the arteries." It's also linked to strokes and heart disease. But outside of the medical professions, people didn't really pay a lot of attention to cholesterol until the 1980s. Suddenly it seemed like *everybody* was worrying about their cholesterol levels—and we learned that anything over 200 mg per deciliter (200mg/dl) was "high" (over 170mg/dl for kids).

So, what *is* cholesterol? It's a waxy, fat-like substance found only in animal products. There are several kinds of cholesterol, two of which you've probably heard about: low density lipoproteins (LDLs) and high density lipoproteins (HDLs). HDL and LDL are not present in foods as HDL and LDL—just cholesterol. Instead, your body decides how much of each form it needs to make and this decision is based on a number of factors—the most obvious being the quality of your diet.

And that's the important point to keep in mind—your body actually *needs* some cholesterol. Not a lot—only about 1.5 grams each day is enough. Cholesterol plays several important roles—it's a key component of the walls of all of your cells, for example, and it's an essential ingredient for your hormones. One of it's most important functions, however, is to carry fats through your bloodstream and out of your body. In fact, it's so important that your body actually *makes* cholesterol, in the liver.

And that last function is something you need to keep in mind, because it's why fat and cholesterol are so closely linked. When you eat a high-fat diet, your body has to move it all through your system. To do this, it steps up production of cholesterol to deal with all that fat. The concern is when an excess of it ends up circulating in the blood, along with fatty material (triglycerides), and these two gradually build up as plaque along the walls of the blood vessels. This plaque causes blockages, restricting the free flow of blood throughout the body. If this build-up occurs in the blood vessels that nourish the heart, it can cause angina or a heart attack. If it occurs in the blood vessels that nourish the brain, it can cause a stroke.

This is where the two different kinds of cholesterol make a difference. LDLs are the ones that circulate through the blood, transporting fats to where they're needed. When they build up to too-high levels, they tend to fall out of the circulating blood and plaster themselves along the walls of your arteries. That's why the LDLs have the reputation of being "the bad guys"—they're the ones responsible for "hardened" arteries, strokes, and heart attacks.

· HDLs, on the other hand, are thought of as "the good guys" because they actually help your body get rid of excess cholesterol and fats in the blood before they can build up along the arterial walls. But they can't do the job alone. In fact, cholesterol can be pretty hard for your body to get rid of. The only way to get excess substances out of the body is through the bowel tract—but cholesterol is very readily reabsorbed if it isn't swept out of the system pretty quickly. That's why dietary fiber is so important. Fiber greatly facilitates your body's efforts to get rid of excess cholesterol.

Most people think of cholesterol as an adult problem—after all, strokes and heart attacks don't happen to kids, right? But the health risks associated with high cholesterol are present for kids, too—and we now know that the longer our bodies act as hosts for high levels of cholesterol, the greater the risk of serious heart disease or stroke in adulthood. What's alarming is that the American Heart Association estimates a full third of our nation's children have high cholesterol levels.

In my practice, I see many overweight kids with high cholesterol—and to be honest, it scares me. These kids are facing all kinds of problems in the years ahead, and these problems will only worsen if they've also got poor eating habits and sedentary lifestyles. The thing is, their parents often seem shocked that this has happened—don't they realize that kids don't get this way by themselves? As parents, it's our responsibility to see to their nutrition and to make sure they stay active. We can't expect our kids—or our teens—to maintain a healthy weight and to value physical activity if we don't teach them by our own example!

So what's the solution? Pay attention to the amount of cholesterol in your family's diet. Go easy on the high-fat, high-cholesterol foods and make sure you're including enough fiber in the diet and enough activity in their day. And if you and your spouse have high cholesterol, make a point of getting your children's cholesterol levels checked regularly. The National Cholesterol Education Program, recognizing that high-cholesterol parents tend to raise high-cholesterol kids, recommends an annual check to make certain that your children's cholesterol levels remain below the 170mg/dl danger zone.

Vitamins

Unlike the nutrients discussed so far, vitamins provide no calories for energy, but are needed by our bodies in order to maintain good health. Your body doesn't make them (except for vitamin D), so you have to get them in your food. You don't need them in large amounts, but a deficiency in any one of them can result in serious problems. The good news is that vitamin deficiencies can be easily avoided, by eating a wide variety of well-balanced meals and snacks. In addition, much of our food supply today is fortified with vitamins.

Scientists have identified a total of 13 vitamins that are essential to good nutrition (see the table, below). Of these, 4 are fat soluble and are found in the fatty foods we eat. The other 9 are water soluble. With the fat-soluble vitamins, too much can be as bad as not enough—they don't dissolve in water, so they can build up in the body tissue and can cause illness or even death.

The 13 Essential Vitamins	
Fat Soluble Vitamins	*Water Soluble Vitamins*
A	B1 (thiamin)
D	B2 (riboflavin)
E	B6 (pyridoxine)
K	B12 (cobalamin)
	Biotin
	Folic Acid
	Niacin
	Pantothenic acid
	C (ascorbic acid)

The Fat-Soluble Vitamins

Fat soluble vitamins are stored in the body until they're needed. Each one plays a specialized role in maintaining your body's functions. Let's look at them one by one.

Vitamin A. Vitamin A is necessary for maintaining the epithelial cells—the cells that make up your skin and line your body's cavities. This vitamin also plays a role in building bone and teeth, and it's essential for good vision. In addition, it helps to strengthen your immune system. Good sources are fish and fish oils, eggs, butter, milk, and cheese.

Your body can also create vitamin A from a substance called beta-carotene, which is found in all pigmented fruits and vegetables. Orange-yellow produce is particularly rich in beta-carotene: carrots, pumpkin, winter squash, cantaloupe, apricots, papaya, and sweet potatoes. The dark-green, leafy veggies are another good source: broccoli, spinach, kale, and collard and turnip greens, for example. In addition to providing the raw material for making vitamin A, beta-carotene is also believed to be an antioxidant. (Antioxidants are nutrients that help to neutralize the oddly charged ions—"free radicals"—that are thought to trigger cancer formation).

Vitamin E. Vitamin E, like beta-carotene, is believed to act as an antioxidant, protecting your body's tissues from damage by strengthening the immune system. It also protects cell membranes. Vitamin E may play a role in lowering the risk of heart disease by increasing HDL ("good cholesterol") and decreasing LDL ("bad cholesterol"). There is also speculation that it may improve blood flow to the brain and slow the progression of Alzheimer's disease.

Good sources of vitamin E are nuts, seeds, wheat germ, vegetable oils, avocados, fish, and whole-grain products. Vitamin E is currently one of the most popular vitamin supplements on the market today. It's antioxidant properties have led some to believe that it will slow down the aging process, making it particularly popular among the elderly. This anti-aging effect, however, has yet to be proven.

Vitamin D. Vitamin D is different from all the other vitamins because it's the only one that your body can make for itself—from sunlight. That's how it got its nickname, "the Sunshine Vitamin." This is helpful, because it isn't found naturally occurring in many foods, but it's very important for good bone development. Without vitamin D, your body can't properly absorb calcium and phosphorus, both of which are needed, as they are the minerals from which bones are formed.

The best natural sources for this vitamin are fatty saltwater fish like herring, mackerel, and salmon. It's also found in liver and in cod liver oil (yuck). Because of its great importance in building strong, healthy bones and helping to reduce the risk of osteoporosis, commercial dairies now fortify their milk with vitamin D.

Vitamin K. Vitamin K is necessary for proper blood clotting —without it, you'd bleed to death. Like vitamin D, it also helps calcium do its work in maintaining strong bones. Good sources of this vitamin are the dark green, leafy vegetables, as well as cauliflower, liver, oats, and soy products.

The Water-Soluble Vitamins

Although there are 9 water-soluble vitamins in all, 8 of them are part of the vitamin B complex. Vitamin C completes the list. The major function of the B vitamins is in the production of energy. They act as catalysts in a variety of ways, as you'll soon see, helping to create energy for doing everything from metabolizing food into energy to creating DNA and RNA, the stuff that our genes are made of.

Vitamin C. Vitamin C, also known as ascorbic acid, is probably the most familiar vitamin for most of us. It's been credited with everything from curing colds to preventing or curing cancer. I'm sure everyone has been told, at one time or another, to "drink your orange juice during cold and flu season." That's because orange juice, as well as many other fruits and vegetables, is a good source of vitamin C. You can get it in citrus fruits, tomatoes, peppers (red, green, and yellow), berries, melons, and tropical fruits (kiwi, papaya, and mango), and in broccoli, cauliflower, and brussel sprouts. Does it really cure the common cold? No one knows for sure, but vitamin C does appear to reduce the duration of cold symptoms.

Vitamin C has a number of other functions as well. First of all, it helps your body make bone, cartilage and tendons. It helps speed the healing of wounds and is important in the formation of red blood cells and certain hormones. It helps your body get rid of cholesterol by carrying it to the liver, where the cholesterol is converted to bile and then excreted. In addition, vitamin C helps process amino acids and functions as an antioxidant.

The B-complex Vitamins. These "Energy Vitamins"—8 in all—are important in a vast array of the body's metabolic processes. Your body only stores one of them, B-12, in the liver. Excess amounts of the others, and of vitamin C, are flushed from the system. The Bs are called energy vitamins because they are important in all aspects of growth, energy production, and metabolism. Here's a brief run-down of each of the Bs:

- *Thiamin (B1).* Thiamin helps the body get energy out of the carbohydrates you consume. Thiamin is present in many grain products, so a B1 deficiency is rare. Best sources of thiamin include lean meats, organ meats, whole grains, fortified cereals, whole grain breads, legumes, wheat germ, and yeast.

- *Riboflavin (B2).* Riboflavin helps support vision and is necessary for healthy skin. Milk, dairy, lean meats, and organ meats are the best sources, but riboflavin is also present in grains, legumes, fortified cereals, some vegetables, and nuts.

- *Niacin.* Niacin helps the body use sugars and fatty acids, and it helps enzymes function properly. It is also believed to play a role in preventing heart disease by helping to lower the blood fats (cholesterol) and triglycerides. However, too much of this vitamin can cause "niacin flush"—your head feels like it's on fire and gets very itchy—the itchiness may even run down your whole body. While probably not dangerous, niacin flush sure is uncomfortable. Still, niacin is important in your diet, and you can get if from liver, poultry, fish, beef, peanut butter, legumes, and whole grains.

- *Pyridoxine (B6).* Vitamin B6 is necessary for making new body cells during periods of growth, so it's especially important in a child's diet. Infants who lack sufficient B6 can suffer inadequate brain and nervous system development, and a deficiency can trigger mental convulsions. No wonder, then, that breast milk is especially high in vitamin B6, or that manufacturers fortify infant cereals with this vitamin.

  B6 also helps make insulin, which regulates blood sugar; hemoglobin for strong red blood cells; and antibodies to fight against infection. Recent research suggests that vitamin B6 may also play a role in the prevention of heart disease by lowering homocysteine levels (homocysteine is an amino acid which, in large amounts, can damage the artery walls). Other good sources of B6 are salmon and herring, wheat germ, bananas, watermelon, lean red meat, chicken, pork, organ meats, whole grains, soy products, and legumes.

- *Cobalamin (B12).* Vitamin B12 is unique because it is the only water soluble vitamin found only in animal products. B12 works closely with folic acid to make red blood cells and prevent anemia, and also has a role in normal nerve function, thought processes, and in the production of neurotransmitters (things like serotonin that help with nerve conduction within the brain). It is also believed to help heart health, like B6, by decreasing homo- cysteine levels.

  But because it's only found in animal products, strict vegans, who shun animal products altogether, run the risk of a B12 deficiency, which causes severe anemia and irreversible nerve damage. Also at risk are people suffering from gastrointestinal diseases, such as Crohn's Disease, because B12 is primarily absorbed in the intestines. Good natural sources of B12 include meat, poultry, seafood, and dairy products. Vegans should definitely supplement with vitamin B12 to make certain that they get enough—about 6 milligrams a day.

- *Folic Acid (folacin).* The role of folic acid in preventing birth defects, and promoting growth during childhood, has often been presented in the media. The recommended daily allowance, which is 400 milligrams, provides enough of this vitamin to avoid the problems of anemia, impaired growth, and, in pregnant women, fetal neural tube defects. Folic acid's most important job is to help the body make new cells, including red blood cells. The best sources of folic acid are green leafy vegetables, dried peas and beans, liver, yeast and yeast breads, and wheat germ. Some fortified cereals, juices, rice, and pasta are enriched with folic acid, too.

- *Biotin.* Biotin helps the body metabolize protein, fat, and carbohydrates for use as energy. It is present in a wide variety of foods, so if you eat a varied diet you probably obtain sufficient amounts of biotin. The best sources are eggs, liver, oatmeal, cereals, yeast, and bakery products made with yeast.

- *Pantothenic Acid.* Pantothenic acid, like biotin, also helps the body metabolize protein, fat, and carbohydrates. It's rare for anyone to develop a deficiency of this vitamin because it's present in so many foods. The flip side is that you can eat too much of it. Excess amounts of pantothenic acid can cause diarrhea and water retention. The best sources of this vitamin are meat, poultry, fish, eggs, whole grain cereals, legumes, and avocados.

Since vitamins are so important, should you consider taking supplements? Well, vitamin C and E supplements wouldn't hurt, as an excess of either seems to rarely have a toxic effect. And for some people on restrictive diets—particularly diets that limit calories and the intake of specific food groups, such as carbohydrates or animal proteins—it may be necessary to take supplements in order to guarantee that you get enough of the B-complex vitamins. Still, your best bet is to follow a healthy eating plan like the one outlined in this book and, for insurance, take a reputable multivitamin and mineral source. This is usually more than enough.

Minerals

Minerals are inorganic elements and, like vitamins, they are calorie free and needed in very small amounts. Although our bodies don't require large quantities of minerals, they are still a vital part of a daily diet.

There are 25 minerals identified to date. Some, like calcium and phosphorus, are used as building blocks; others act as catalysts in a number of different chemical processes in the body; and others, like sodium and chloride, act on their own, as electrolytes, to perform special functions, such as regulating body temperature, fluid balance and nerve impulses. In the section that follows you'll find an explanation of several of the minerals that are most important in maintaining strong, healthy bodies.

The Building Blocks: Calcium and Phosphorus. As a nation, we have progressively cut back on our calcium intake over the years—largely because we tend to reach for a soda instead of pouring a glass of milk. This is particularly unfortunate for our children, because approximately 90 percent of the adult skeleton is formed before the age of 17, and 60 percent of the body's bone mass is finalized during puberty. Without an adequate supply of calcium, our children's bodies simply can't produce enough healthy bone, and they wind up with an increased risk of osteoporosis as young adults.

Calcium and phosphorus are the most abundant minerals in the human body, and they're concentrated in your bones and teeth: over 95 percent of the body's calcium and 89 percent of its phosphorus can be found there. These 2 minerals also play a role in muscle contraction and the conduction of nerve impulses.

Calcium is also important elsewhere in the body, working with other nutrients in a number of different ways. For example, it helps vitamin K in promoting blood clotting. And, together with phosphorus and certain electrolytes, it plays an important role in muscle contraction and nerve conduction. Calcium is also believed to play a role in preventing high blood pressure by competing with sodium in some way that is, as yet, not fully understood.

Your calcium needs change over the course of your lifetime. The best source of calcium is from low-fat milk and other dairy products—and if they're fortified with vitamin D and magnesium, the calcium they contain will be more efficiently absorbed by the body. You can also get calcium from sardines with bone, salmon, shrimp, tofu, fortified soy and rice milk, and almonds. You can get calcium from vegetables, too, but this is a less efficient source, in part because vegetable-derived calcium is less readily absorbed by the body.

Most healthcare professionals recommend a calcium supplement, particularly for young adolescent and adult females, because they face special risks later on in life. If you're looking for a supplement, avoid those that are made from "natural" oyster shell, bone meal, or dolomite—they're bogus and may contain lead. Check the labels and stick to reputable supplements of calcium carbonate or calcium citrate.

Magnesium. Like calcium and phosphorus, most of your body's magnesium is found in the bone. That's because magnesium works side by side with calcium and phosphorus in the formation and maintenance of bones and teeth. Magnesium also works with them to regulate blood pressure, body temperature, nerve transmission, and muscle contraction. It also helps your body absorb calcium and utilize zinc.

Recently, there has been some speculation that people with Type 2 diabetes mellitus and even glucose intolerance (high blood sugar levels, which often precedes Type 2 diabetes), may suffer from a magnesium deficiency. In other words, individuals who are deficient in magnesium tend to have poor control over their blood sugar levels.

A healthy diet provides 400 milligrams of magnesium a day, which you can get from whole grains, dried beans, nuts, fruits, green veggies, seafood, honey, molasses, and—chocolate! If you're not getting enough in the foods you eat, most multi-vitamin tablets that include minerals will help out. If you choose a magnesium supplement, look for one that combines calcium as well, at a ratio of about 2 to 1, calcium to magnesium.

Sodium, Potassium, and Chloride. Sodium, potassium, and chloride act as electrolytes in the body. An electrolyte is an ion with an electrical charge. These substances are important because, when they're dissolved in water, they break apart and conduct electrical charges that are vital for muscular contractions and nerve impulses. They are also important in regulating your body's temperature and fluid balance.

Sodium and chloride are common in every household—they're what table salt is made of. Unfortunately, most people consume much more sodium chloride than they need, and typically more than they realize. A single teaspoon of salt contains 2,000 milligrams of sodium alone. In addition, most processed and packaged foods have large amounts of both sodium and chloride, as they are both present in a large majority of the preservatives used by the food processing industry.

It's believed that sodium increases blood pressure, whereas potassium, like calcium, seems to have the opposite effect—in part because it helps the body to get rid of excess sodium. Good sources of potassium include bananas, citrus fruits, potatoes, tomatoes, cantaloupe, lean meats, bran, and oats.

Iron. Iron is extremely important during periods of rapid growth, which is basically throughout childhood and adolescence and well into the early adult years. It plays a key role in the formation of red blood cells, and especially in the transportation of oxygen to the brain and muscles. The iron in the blood attaches to oxygen atoms, carrying them throughout the body and releasing them where they're needed. Children who fail to get adequate iron can suffer impaired development of the brain and it's cognitive function. Adults who lack sufficient iron suffer from anemia, with symptoms of fatigue, lethargy, headaches, lack of the ability to concentrate, and/or shortness of breath.

It's particularly important that girls and young women get adequate iron in their daily diet. With the onset of puberty, iron loss through the monthly menstrual flow can seriously deplete a girl's iron supply. Yet iron is the one mineral most likely to be lacking in a young person's diet, and nearly 75 percent of all girls aged 12 to 19 do not get the recommended amount of 18 mg of iron each day. Compounding the problem is society's infatuation with thinness. Many young women respond to this social pressure by reducing their intake of beef and dairy products because they're under the false impression that these food groups are "fattening." The truth is, they're not—but they are two of the best sources of iron and calcium, respectively.

Iron comes in two forms: heme and non-heme. Heme iron is the more readily absorbed form. It's found in animal products, especially beef and livers, which is why I usually recommend that parents include 2 to 3 servings of beef in their children's weekly diet. Non-heme iron, which is found in dark green, leafy vegetables like spinach and kale, is not as easily absorbed by the body as heme iron, but you can increase it's absorption by adding a vitamin C source, such as citrus fruits or tomatoes to the meal. For example, if you put lemon or tomato sauce on your spinach, or follow the meal with an orange for dessert, you will increase your body's ability to absorb the iron. Other sources of non-heme iron include dried fruits, such as raisins, prunes, and apricots, dried peas and beans, soybeans, wheat germ, rolled oats, cherry juice, blackstrap molasses, and shredded wheat.

Even if you eat foods high in heme, you may still not be absorbing the iron as efficiently as you should, because certain substances in our food supply compete with iron for absorption—and iron often loses the competition! This is especially true if you drink coffee or tea or take antacids. The caffeine in coffee, the tannins in tea, and the magnesium in antacids each reduce the body's ability to absorb iron by competing with it. Excessive amounts of milk can also reduce iron absorption. The best thing is to avoid these items when you're eating an iron-rich meal. In other words, serve vegetable juice or diluted fruit juice instead of milk with the meal. And for you adults, no coffee immediately after a dinner of spinach and noodles. Wait an hour or so, to allow your body to absorb the iron and digest the food first, and then have your coffee or tea.

Iron supplements are a good idea—especially for adolescent and teenage girls and premenopausal women, all of whom are at greater risk of developing anemia (from iron deficiency) due to their monthly menstrual flow. But taking an iron pill by itself can cause constipation for some, which is why I always recommend that pre-menopausal women take a multi-vitamin with iron. Men and postmenopausal women, however, should NOT take a multi-vitamin or mineral containing iron, unless advised to do so by their doctor, as the most recent research suggests that too much iron can cause heart disease.

Zinc. Zinc is found in every tissue in the body. It plays a major role in energy metabolism and in the making of protein. It's also important for taste and smell perception, wound healing, physical growth, and sexual maturation. Zinc may also have a role with vitamin C in fighting off or lessening the severity of colds, and it may help prevent heart disease by keeping blood vessels healthy. Adults need about 15 milligrams of zinc a day, and most adults get enough zinc in their regular diets because it's found in a lot of different foods: lean beef, egg yolk, oysters, liver, fish, lamb, and pork, as well as in whole grain products, sesame and sunflower seeds, soybeans, mushrooms, and brewer's yeast.

Children, however, do run the risk of a zinc deficiency. This shouldn't be too surprising—one look at the list above shows clearly that the majority of zinc-rich foods are not your typical children's fare. It's estimated that only 20 percent of children between the ages of 1 and 3, and only 50 percent of children aged 4 to 6, get the full recommended allowance of zinc each day. But supplementing may not be the answer, because excessive zinc can be dangerous—doses over 50 milligrams can weaken the immune system, which would leave your child more susceptible to disease. Yet another good reason it's better to choose whole grain products for your family.

Chromium. Chromium helps the body metabolize carbohydrates, which in turn influence blood sugar levels and the production of energy. It seems to do this by helping insulin "push" glucose (blood sugar) into the cells, making the body more energy efficient. Because of this function, it is thought that chromium may help those with glucose intolerance and Type 1 and Type 2 diabetes control their blood sugar (and thus, help manage their diabetes better). Natural sources of chromium are liver, whole grains, peanuts, brewer's yeast, animal protein, cheese, mushrooms, spinach, black pepper, oranges, and even wine and beer.

Some believe chromium is lost when we eat simple sugars, and that a deficiency of chromium will lead to sugar cravings. This is the logic behind the health food stores that push chromium as a weight loss and energy supplement. The research is still very controversial and, as yet, inconclusive. As of September 1997, the FDA has cracked down on some of the more extravagant claims of supplement manufacturers. Manufacturers of chromium piccolinate supplements can no longer claim that their product will burn fat, cause weight loss, increase muscle mass, reduce serum cholesterol, regulate blood sugar levels, or fight diabetes mellitus.

Selenium. is becoming more and more recognized as an important mineral, although it is still not fully understood. It has gained media attention because it is one of the minerals that may be destroyed as agricultural land is overused and the soils are depleted. Among selenium's benefits for the body is its function as an antioxidant, keeping the immune system strong, and working with vitamin C to help prevent the cellular damage that often results in cancer. It is also involved in normal growth and development and is needed to maintain tissue elasticity. Natural sources of selenium are wheat bran and wheat germ, brewer's yeast, whole grains, tuna, herring, broccoli, onions, and mushrooms.

Is our natural supply of selenium being depleted, as some claim? No one seems to know for sure, so a supplement might be a good idea. However, selenium is one of those nutrients that can be toxic if you get too much—and anything over 200 milligrams a day is too much! 55 milligrams a day is more appropriate.

BUT THAT'S NOT ALL. . .

By now you've got a solid grasp of the basics of nutrition, but there are some special considerations you should keep in mind before moving on to the next chapters. These special considerations have to do with the way that foods have been altered in recent times, and the way our tastes have been shaped by some pretty aggressive marketing—marketing that is more interested in building profits than in providing healthful foods.

Sugar substitutes

When the public became aware of the empty calories in refined sugar, there was a big demand for a substitute that would give us that sweet taste we crave without all those empty calories. The result was a whole raft of products, from saccharine to aspartame and, more recently, sucralose. Unfortunately, although most studies show they are safe in moderate amounts, none of these studies are done with kids (it's against the law to test products on kids or pregnant women), so there is really very little known about the effects of these substitutes on growth. The manufacturers may try to claim that they're safe, but there's no evidence to support this assertion. In my personal opinion, sugar substitutes should *not* be a part of a growing child's intake.

Saccharine. Saccharine—today marketed under the name of Sweet N Low—has been used for many, many years. In it's earliest form it came in tiny tablets, but now you can get it in granulated and liquid form as well. After an early period of approval, it was later suspected of causing cancer, but when insufficient scientific evidence of carcinogens were found, it was re-approved by the FDA. While it's still around, many of the products initially sweetened with saccharine are now using the newer substitutes, aspartame and sucralose.

Aspartame. Aspartame, better known as Nutrasweet and sold under the brand name Equal, has been in our food supply since 1981. It's a combination of 2 amino acids, bonded together. While it's called safe by the FDA, the American Diabetes Association, and the World Health Organization, there's a troubling problem. One of its amino acids is phenylalanine, and a small minority of people are born without the enzyme to digest this substance. For these people, the phenylalanine builds up in the blood and can cause brain damage—a condition known as phenylketonuria. That's why there's a warning on products containing aspartame. A small percentage of people also appear to have a sensitivity to aspartame, claiming that it gives them headaches. Other more vigilant groups have gone so far as to blame it for causing multiple sclerosis, Alzheimer's, and brain tumors, but there is really no scientific evidence to support these claims, and therefore it remains approved for use.

Sucralose. This is the newest of the artificial sweeteners on the general market. According to the manufacturer, Sucralose, sold under the brand name Splenda, is made from sugar through a multi-step, patented chemical process that alters the sugar molecule. It has no calories because this alteration makes it pass thru the body essentially unchanged—the body doesn't digest it or absorb it.

Other sweeteners. There's a bunch of sweeteners called hydrogenated starch hydrosylates (HSHs) that have no nutritional value to speak of. Marketed under the names of Sorbitol, Xylitol, and Manitol, they're made of sugars to which hydrogen has been added. They look like corn syrup but function like artificial sweeteners. These products are not as sweet as sugar, and *all* of them have a laxative effect if consumed in excess —say, if you consumed ten pieces of "sugar free" candy or gum. And then there's Stevia, an herb from Paraguay (*Stevia rebundiana*). Stevia is typically found in health food stores, where it's marketed as a "natural" sweetener. It's 200 to 300 times sweeter than sucrose but has no calories. It's believed to be safe for human consumption and has been used in other countries for many years. It has a slight licorice taste and aftertaste.

Fat "Substitutes"

Lots of people think of margarine and other oleo products as fat "substitutes." That's usually not the case. It's true that you can substitute margarine for butter, but it's still fat. Margarine was initially developed during the World War II era to get around a butter shortage. The early product was a white, lard-like lump and was often sold with a packet of yellow dye that could be mixed in to make it look more like the "real thing." Since then there have been many new fat "substitute" products. Here are some of the more widely used ones out there:

Trans fatty acids. This includes almost all of today's margarines. Trans fat is made by hydrogenating (adding a hydrogen molecule to) vegetable oil, which hardens the oil to make it more solid and gives it a longer shelf life. Margarine was initially thought to be healthier than butter, because it did not contain the cholesterol and saturated fats found in the animal based butter. However, the over-hydrogenation process used to make margarine results in a fat that's just as bad for the heart as the saturated fat and cholesterol it was supposed to replace. Trans-fats are now know to raise "bad" cholesterol—LDLs—and may even decrease the HDLs ("good" cholesterol)!

Some scientists even believe that trans fats may be responsible for thousands of heart disease-related deaths each year. This is definitely possible when you think about how many people switched to margarine from butter over the past 10 years. Unfortunately, these fats are now found in everything from processed snacks and bakery products to flavored rice and pasta mixes, and the label never says "trans fat." You can, however, identify the product by checking the list of ingredients: just look for the words "hydrogenated" or "partially hydrogenated" and avoid these foods as much as possible.

Olestra (fake fat). Olestra is a chemical fat substitute that cannot be absorbed or digested by the human body. Unfortunately, it doesn't allow your body to absorb fat-soluble vitamins, either. And, as you learned in Chapter 3, many people experience some pretty unpleasant side effects from it. It's typically used in crunchy snack foods—the WOW brand of potato chips is an Olestra-based product. The problem is that kids are big fans of crunchy junk foods, but they should *not* be eating foods with olestra. Sure, it had to pass FDA standards for safety—but the tests were *never* done on kids (remember: testing on kids is against the law), so nobody has a clue as to how dangerous it might be for them. Given that it blocks the absorption of essential fat soluble vitamins, it's potentially dangerous for a growing child. I feel so strongly about this that when I've actually spotted kids eating those WOW chips, you can believe I said something to their parents about it!

But the biggest problem with these products is the false sense of security they give. People have been led to believe that if something's "fat-free" they can eat all they want. The same thing holds true for the "sugar-free" products out there. The problem is that "fat-free" foods are usually loaded with sugar, and "sugar-free" foods are usually high in fat! My philosophy is simple: skip the labels that say "free" and eat the regular variety. Just learn to eat a reasonable portion of it.

Caffeine

You may be wondering why I'm mentioning caffeine here. Well, believe it or not, you—and your kids—are probably getting a lot of caffeine in your diet, even if *nobody* in your household drinks coffee. It's the most widely consumed psychoactive substance (stimulant) in the world, according to Christian Millman, whose article "The Buzz on Soft Drinks and Caffeine" appears on the Discovery.com Website. Most parents wouldn't let their young kids drink a cup of coffee, never mind drinking it by the pot full, but they think nothing of letting a child order a super-sized Coke or Pepsi at the local fast-food restaurant. But that soft drink is just *loaded* with caffeine.

So is chocolate! We've spent a lot of time over the past couple of decades talking about how kids should avoid sugar because the sugar rush can jazz them up so much, but we never even mentioned the caffeine buzz they're getting from that chocolate-based candy bar!

Caffeine-based soft drinks are a particular problem because kids reach for them when they're feeling thirsty, without realizing that the caffeine can actually hasten dehydration. It's a diuretic, which means that it steps up urine production, rapidly ridding the body of much needed water. It's far better to get your children used to reaching for plain water when they want to quench their thirst.

Caffeine, whether it's in a soft drink, a cup of coffee or tea, a chocolate candy bar, or anything else, is immediately absorbed into the bloodstream. In adults it has the potential to wreak havoc on the central nervous system, causing headaches, nervousness, anxiety, insomnia, digestive problems, muscle twitching, an altered heart rate, and so on. Obviously, children are even more vulnerable to its effects. In addition, in children caffeine adds the danger of interfering with their bodies' absorption of calcium and iron!

BODIES IN MOTION 6

$\mathcal{W}$ellness requires physical activity, just as much as it requires healthy eating. And although lots of health clubs for fitness-minded adults are springing up everywhere, and exercise videos led by everybody from Jane Fonda to Richard Simmons are being released everyday, very little attention is paid to our kids' need for exercise. Maybe we figure they're getting enough exercise just by *being* kids!

But here's an eye-opening revelation and a very sobering thought: Even though we envision our kids as bubbling with energy, unable to sit still, the reality is that many children lack plain, old- fashioned playtime in their days. All that activity we think they're getting? They're *not!* And this has some serious long-term consequences for their health. In fact, researchers are now beginning to show that the biggest contributing factor to childhood obesity (and adult obesity as well) is *inactivity*!

The problem has become so great that the surgeon general has declared inactivity as a risk factor for heart disease—giving it the same weight as smoking and eating a high-fat diet! It's for this reason that, in my practice, I teach that even the most nutritious diet in the world is not enough to help our kids build strong, healthy bodies. They need the same emphasis given to regular, daily physical activity, too.

WHO TOOK THE FUN OUT OF BEING A KID?!

Childhood has traditionally been "prime time" for active play. But the reality is that activity, like so much else, has become a luxury that many can't afford. Children from wealthier backgrounds are able to afford structured regimens of dance lessons, soccer practice, and other physical outlets for all their energy, so long as their parents are willing and able to chauffeur them around.

Less privileged children often live latchkey lives. Their parents can't afford the luxury of relying on a single income, and sometimes there's only one wage earner in the house to begin with. They surely can't afford an au pair or a sitter and, in our transient society, they don't have nearby friends and relatives who are capable or willing to fill in the gaps. So their kids are trapped in their houses or apartments after school, plopped in front of a TV or VCR.

But even privileged children enrolled in lessons are missing something pretty important: unstructured, spontaneous, silly play. Unstructured play is an important part of childhood development. It lets kids test their limits without judgment. It lets them explore new territories without boundaries. And believe it or not, all of this silly, spontaneous fun builds self-confidence. Contrast this with worrying about making the team, performing well enough to get into the game, and keeping proud Mom and Dad happy by hitting a home run or making the winning goal.

Plain Old Playtime

True play offers more than just activity. Because it is unstructured and uncontrolled, it lets kids be kids. It lets them imagine—and conquer—new challenges, which helps build character and self-confidence. When they see their accomplishments —climbing trees or monkey bars, jumping on one foot while playing hop scotch, racing to the corner against friends—they can feel good about themselves without a referee or judge criticizing their performance. They can have fun without worrying about whether or not they're living up to grown-up expectations.

Play—that is, play with other kids—also fosters social growth. Kids learn to share, learn to deal with personality differences, learn to accommodate the individual traits of others. In short, they learn how to get along in and with the world. Kids who feel good about themselves are usually more outgoing and more interested in learning about the world around them. Even more introverted children benefit immensely from interacting with other children. There is a certain magic that evolves when children play together. The more extroverted kids usually make an effort to involve everyone in their fun, which helps the shy children build their social etiquette, teaching them how to interact with a variety of personalities. They learn how to get along well with others and, as they build self-assurance, they learn how to resist peer pressure, too.

Structured play lets kids be active, but it's usually controlled by adults. That means that the children don't usually have a chance to learn how to resolve problems among themselves—the grown-ups are all too ready to get into the middle of a dispute or call a time-out. That's not an entirely bad thing—we all want to step in and protect our kids from feeling sad or getting hurt—but if adults are always in charge, kids never learn how to handle problems on their own. And let's face it, everyone eventually faces disappointment and unexpected challenges in their lives. There's nothing wrong with allowing kids to experience these negative situations—it's better they learn to deal with different emotions now, early on, then to allow them to be rudely awakened at a much older age.

Maybe we need to turn back the hands of time and just let kids be kids. Let them rediscover the old-fashioned joy of hopscotch, hide and seek, jumping rope . . . or just plain being silly. Organized activities like sports training and dance class, if your budget allows it, are certainly beneficial, but they're no substitute for pure, unadulterated playtime. The key: work to create a healthy balance between the two.

While we're on the subject of "turning back time," here's something you could try that will help your kids come up with more active or stimulating ways of amusing themselves. One night a month, pretend there's no electricity. (Okay, you can turn on the lights, but *that's all!*) No TV, no computer and no battery operated GameBoys either—you have to spend the entire evening doing things that do not require electricity. A good old-fashioned game of *Monopoly* or *Twister* would be good choices if you're staying indoors. Reading together, or even playing charades can be fun. Otherwise, when the great outdoors beckons—go for it! (I sometimes use a "no TV for a day" rule when my son seems pushed to his limits and needs an attitude change. It works wonders.)

Where Have all the Playgrounds Gone?

Let's face it, parents today are overbooked and overburdened. We're a society in overdrive, with less and less free time for doing the things we really want to do—like playing with our kids. With all this pressure, we typically put our families—and even our own health—on the back-burner, while we concentrate on fulfilling the practical demands of our jobs. But that's not the only reason physical activity has taken a back-seat in our lives and the lives of our kids.

Equally responsible for our lack of physical activity is society at large. The decisions of our policy makers have had a major impact on our ability to get active and *stay* active. If you don't believe me, check out this list of just *some* of the ways that modern life works against our kids' physical fitness.

1. **No place to play**. The boom in land development began in the 1960s and then really went out of control in the 1980s. Suddenly, vacant land was worth a fortune, and the empty lots and undeveloped woodlands of our childhood began to disappear under the bulldozer's blade. The demand for land is now so strong that houses are no longer built on large lots with nice yards—instead, they get a postage-stamp sized area of grass around them, all the better to squeeze a few more units into the development. Don't believe me? Go visit the neighborhood you grew up in and see for yourself. How many new things have been built up there during the last 5, 10, or 15 years?

   And all this development means that children have less and less land to play on. But what's the alternative? The same gyms and health clubs that actively court adult members rarely let kids under 16 in to use the facilities—mainly due to legal liability issues should the kids get hurt. Most of them don't even provide play areas for kids to frequent while their parents are working out, either.

2. **Official policies that make our communities unsafe.** We've already talked about how many people no longer feel safe in their neighborhoods. Sure, some of it is the inevitable consequence of our society's mobility—it's hard to put down roots these days when we're constantly on the

move due to the demands of our jobs. But our local officials haven't helped, either. For example, during the 1980s, a lot of budget-cutters decided to cope with high energy costs by cutting back on street lighting. In some areas, they opted to light alternate street lamps. In others, they shut them down completely! So now, once Daylight Savings Time hits in October, many communities are dark as early as 5 or 6 PM—too dark for kids to go outside to play after dinner!

3. **Cutbacks in school activity and sports programs**. Whatever happened to daily gym class and the President's Council on Physical Fitness challenges we used to have in school? As recently as the 1970s, public schools required all of their students to take physical education classes 5 days a week—from the elementary grades through high school —and this was in addition to the 2 daily recess periods that elementary school kids had outdoors on the playground. If a child failed physical education due to lack of participation or poor performance, they also failed academically for the year—even if they had straight A's in their other classes!

   When I was a child, we participated in everything from archery and baseball to track and field. Looking back, I realize this was a wonderful thing. Physical education exposed us to a wide array of activities, giving us the opportunity to see what we enjoyed and discover what we were good at.

   Back then, many schools also had strong after- school sports programs, and students could choose among alternatives ranging from baseball, basketball, and football to track, cheerleading, and the marching band! I know that at least 75 percent of the students in my school were involved in such programs. Now, however, few schools offer extracurricular activities of any kind, and most have dramatically cut back their physical education classes, as well, for lack of funds. Parents who wish to expose their children to the same enjoyment of sports must enroll them in private lessons or recreational teams sponsored by their towns. Kids whose parents can't afford to or who lack the time to participate—or who don't make the "cut"—are left out in the cold.

In generations past, educators understood what researchers have demonstrated in study after study: that physical health and physical fitness is important for optimal mental performance. In fact, one recent study compared kids who got 5 hours of vigorous activity per week with those who had only 2 hours per week. The result: the first group showed greater improvement in their endurance and strength, as you'd expect, but they *also* showed greater improvement in their language, math, science, and English skills as well! Today, however, schools seem to ignore this important truth—they treat physical activity as a luxury, not a necessity, so they're quick to cut sports and exercise out of the school day. If we truly care about giving our children the best possible advantages in both their health *and* their educational development, we need to get physical activity back into our schools!

4.   **Restricting access to creative opportunities.** Some of the best childhood play—for promoting fitness and for building strong, healthy character and personalities— isn't found in sports. It's in the unstructured, spontaneous, creative play that children initiate on their own. But the opportunity for creative play has become hard to come by. In many communities, education reformers have given up on the traditional public schools—where most of our kids spend their days—and have set up magnet schools and gifted-student programs.

This sounded like a good idea at the time. Kids compete for places in these programs, so you can be pretty sure that they're highly motivated. But over the past couple of decades, we've discovered a few unpleasant consequences of this trend. For example, the competition to get in—and the burden of maintaining high enough grades to stay in—have added tons of toxic stress to our kids' lives. And, of course, there are all those kids who *don't* get in (the majority!)—where are their opportunities for creativity? Students who are academically average or even below-average have a right to creative expression, too!

The only alternative to these "special" programs is, for most kids, a private school. But the tuition charged at private schools puts this option out of reach for most families. So, basically, we're dividing our kids into 2 categories—the favored few who can get access to stimulating, creative opportunities, and the vast majority who cannot. But *all* our children need the opportunity to learn how their bodies move, what to do to improve their abilities, how to physically and emotionally interact with others, and all the other benefits that go into what we used to call "good sportsmanship." These lessons are important to everybody, not just to the few who qualify for or can afford special programs.

So What do Kids Really Need?

Presidents Dwight D. Eisenhower and John F. Kennedy knew the value of physical activity. Eisenhower inaugurated the President's Council on Physical Fitness in the 1950s, and Kennedy challenged the public schools to get the nation's children involved in a regular program of exercise. Kennedy was concerned that "we have become more and more not a nation of athletes, but a nation of spectators." And when it comes to recognizing the importance of fitness for educational excellence, here's what Kennedy had to say on the subject:

> Physical fitness is not only one of the most important keys to a healthy body, it is the basis of dynamic and creative intellectual activity. Intelligence and skill can only function at the peak of their capacity when the body is strong. Hardy spirits and tough minds usually inhabit sound bodies.

We're not talking about sculpting bulging biceps or a set of "six-pack abs" here. Our concern is with physical fitness—getting enough exercise so that the body is able to perform its daily tasks without becoming exhausted, and with enough additional energy left over to enjoy all that life has to offer. The beauty of exercising for fitness is that it involves much more than just the muscles—it strengthens the heart, the lungs and the mind, as well.

Physical fitness is not the same thing as training to become a world-class athlete. Hard-core training is neither necessary nor appropriate for most kids. They don't need to join a gym or work out

on special exercise equipment. They *do*, however, need to participate in at least some type of rigorous activity for about 30 to 60
minutes in duration, 3 to 5 times a week—though ideally the goal
is every day. Come to think of it, that's not a bad objective for people of *any* age to strive for.

So, what should you be aiming for when you're trying to encourage your kids to get—and stay—physically active? That depends on your child. When it comes to physical activity, there's a
wide range of variation even among kids of the same age—some
have highly developed stamina, fine-motor skills, concentration,
and physical courage. Others of the same age may be more timid,
less coordinated, or more easily distracted. But *all* of them will
benefit from some form of regular, vigorous activity.

The American Alliance for Health, Physical Education, Recreation, and Dance (AAHPERD) is the only national-level organization dedicated to improving public awareness about the basic
importance of sports, recreation, and physical education. Of its 6
divisions, the largest is the National Association for Sport and
Physical Education (NASPE). According to NASPE, all elementary
school children should optimally get a good 60 minutes or more of
physical activity *every single day*. Here's the full list of their guidelines for physical fitness:

- At least 60 minutes a day of developmentally appropriate
  activities.

- Extended periods of inactivity are not appropriate for normal,
  healthy children. (This goal is particularly hard for most of our
  kids to meet. They end up sitting in school for up to 8 hours each
  weekday, plus a half-hour or more riding the bus back and
  forth, plus a couple of hours of homework, topped off by a couple of hours spent in front of the TV! This is NOT a good scenario for a growing child, but this is a typical day for far too
  many of our kids.)

- A variety of physical activities of various intensity levels are recommended. For example, some could be in 15 minute spurts of
  intense activity, whereas others, of lesser intensity, such as walking or bicycling, could last longer.

Most major fitness organizations note that young children
(under 8), while they're inherently active, have shorter attention
spans compared to adolescents and adults. To keep them interested,

they need a wide variety of activities and experiences—and that variety also helps them to discover more about their own abilities and interests. It's also important to recognize that kids are most likely to enjoy physical activity if family members and friends also participate. This is no different from adults who prefer the company of others in a fitness center environment, as opposed to being alone. Exercise, taught early, can easily become a habit. This is a habit well worth cultivating.

But these recommendations come with precautions. Parents who wish to encourage physical activity in their children are strongly urged to avoid pressuring your children to excel in sports and games. This performance pressure only makes the event stressful and takes all the fun out of it. When winning is treated as the only reason for playing, all it takes is one defeat to turn a child away from ever trying again. It's much better to teach your child that "It's not whether you win or lose, it's whether you had fun with your teammates."

And here's one last warning: No matter how important physical fitness is, there is a real danger of getting too much of a good thing, particularly with young, growing children. Excessive exercise can in fact cause undue stress on a child's system! In particular, the growth plates in the bones—areas where further development occurs—are still coming together, even in older kids who look physically mature. In fact, bone growth isn't complete until age 18 for girls and age 19 for boys. And for younger children (8 years old or younger) the central nervous system is still under development, too—so little kids don't have the muscle control they'd need to protect themselves. In other words, if your kids go overboard in exercising, they can wind up with muscle injury, dehydration, and even decreased immune-system function.

The Physical Benefits of Fitness

Keeping trim. We all know that exercise burns calories—that's why all reputable weight loss programs and major health organizations strongly encourage you to get active every day. But burning calories during exercise is only a very small part of the story. In addition, regular physical activity increases the body's metabolic rate by promoting muscle development—and a higher metabolic rate means that the body will naturally burn more calories. In fact, it's estimated that with each pound of muscle you develop, your body will burn at least 35 extra calories each day. Do the math—one additional pound of muscle will result in approximately 12,775 extra calories burned each year! And exercise gives you stronger muscles, greater endurance, more flexibility, and pumps up your energy level.

Building up the bones. Regular exercise is also important for building strong bones. Walking, running, and dancing—all activities that involve weight-bearing exercise—help the body reinforce the skeletal system. This, in turn, contributes to the development of good posture, decreases the risk of injury and helps prevent osteoporosis.

Exercises the insides, too. Regular physical exercise strengthens more than just the obvious muscle groups. Keep in mind that the body's internal organs—including the brain, liver, kidney, and lungs—are muscles too. Activity also gives the heart and endocrine system a work-out. It strengthens the heart and helps to lower the heart rate and blood pressure. It also improves the functioning of the immune and digestive systems and enhances circulation, improving the delivery of oxygen throughout the body. It even helps the body's cells become more receptive to insulin, which helps prevent Type 2 diabetes mellitus—the type associated with being overweight!

Fitness and Emotional Health

Exercise improves emotional health, too. Part of this comes from purely physiological factors—exercise increases endorphin and adrenaline production, the naturally occurring substances in the body that produce what's known as the "runner's high." These substances are your body's own, naturally occurring mood enhancers, and when they're released they help combat feelings of depression and lethargy. Why? Because when you're up and moving, you typically feel better about yourself. And the simple fact that you're out and about makes you more outgoing, too!

And while we're on the subject, think about this: physical activity has been shown time and again to help reduce physical and emotional stress. And by improving circulation and promoting blood flow to the brain, it helps stimulate the mind—the link between physical activity and improved intellectual performance is now undisputed. Exercise even helps build self esteem! When kids—and even adults—succeed at a physical challenge, the sense of mastery they feel carries over into all other aspects of their self image!

Lifelong Benefits

Getting into the habit of regular exercise at an early age has a tremendous benefit throughout life. In fact, experts believe that for every hour of exercise, a person can gain a 2-hour increase in life span! With these benefits, it's obviously a good idea to make exercise an important part of any child's life. And it really *is* never too late to start. In most circumstances, even a life-long couch potato can reap the same rewards from fitness as someone who has been exercising for years. That said, the sooner you begin, the healthier you will be! So what are you waiting for? No more excuses!

GETTING WITH THE PROGRAM

How can you make sure that your child is getting enough real exercise in their lives? In an ideal world, all kids would have a neighborhood of pals to play with, allowing them to obtain all of the activity their growing bodies required, just by being outside. But there are far too many children who don't live in such ideal surroundings.

Kids Will Be Kids

If you're fortunate enough to live in an area where kids still have an opportunity to indulge in self-directed play, count yourself lucky. Most kids really *do* like to be active, particularly when they're still quite young, and they all like to play outside, although sometimes you have to insist that they "turn off the TV and go out to play!" And once you do manage to get them outside, they don't need lots of toys to keep them active—kids have great imaginations and can turn even the most insignificant objects into a playground of fun.

When my son, Alexander, was in pre-school, he had more fun playing outside "like a psycho-child" (getting silly), than he did with all of his toys! Kids love tag, hide-and-seek, exploring, climbing, and digging in the dirt. Sure they'll get dirty, and they'll probably pick up a bump and bruise or two, but that's all part of growing up too! Children rarely have fears of getting hurt when they're young—it's typically an over-protective parent or caretaker that instills them with a fear that they may fall and hurt themselves.

Older kids can still enjoy this kind of silly play. My son, now 7 years old, certainly does. But he's also becoming more interested in exploring the world and testing his capabilities. Like most kids his age, he enjoys bikes, skates, scooters—anything that lets him expand his horizons a little. He's also more interested in team sports and competition—hockey and judo are his favorites. But even with older kids, toys and equipment aren't all that important as long as they've got space and opportunities to get creative and active. Trees invite climbing, streams invite wading. Snow means snow forts and snowball fights and sledding down hills—and if you don't have a sled, the lid of a garbage can will do in a pinch.

The beauty of activity during the young years is that it teaches kids to have fun using their bodies. Activity becomes something they appreciate for its own sake. And this can be really important when they get into their teen years, and they suddenly discover that they're too "cool" for all the silly games of childhood. A teen who has learned early in life that exercise is fun and feels good is liable to find ways to keep active, and will often carry the commitment to exercise into their adult life, too. This is especially important for girls. Girls between the ages of 12 to 16 are statistically the least active group of kids. The unfortunate irony is that this is also a really crucial stage—it's the turning point that often determines whether a child will become active or sedentary as an adult!

A Fitness Program that Fits

The reality is that many children lack easy access to opportunities for physical activity. For these kids, it is up to the parents to find alternatives. Fortunately, many communities do provide opportunities—you just have to find them. Start by looking in the community section of your local newspaper or going online to find your town or county's Web page. You can also contact your town's Parks and Recreation Department, your local Police Athletic League (PAL), Boys and Girls Clubs, Jewish Community Centers, your local Y. And don't forget to check out the Yellow

Pages for structured lessons in dance and martial arts. Once you start looking, you'll see that there are a number of options to choose from. Many (but not all) are free or require only modest amounts of money for uniforms or other incidentals. Finally, you can go the "do it yourself" route—establishing and supervising activities on your own or with other interested parents.

But not all exercise programs are created equal. You want to investigate before signing your child up. A good exercise program should provide for a solid 30 to 60 minutes of supervised activity, led by a qualified professional who knows the activity and can interact well with children. The program should be scheduled at least 3 times a week and it should combine a variety of activities, giving kids the chance to explore their capabilities, skills, and limits while discovering what they enjoy most. After all, kids are most likely to stay with a program if it's fun. If you can't find a program that offers a 3-times a week schedule (and sadly, that's most of them), consider signing your child up for more than one activity. Alternatively, you can get together with other interested parents and schedule your own "extra" practice session.

And it's best if the program is adaptable to both indoors and outdoors, so bad weather doesn't have to mean canceling the day's exercise—although this is not always feasible for some activities. Finally, the bulk of the time should be devoted to actual play, instead of taking up a lot of time with setting up equipment, changing into exercise clothes, or talking about the day's activities.

Team Players

Another option is to sign your child up for a local team— from Little League to soccer to swimming. There are lots of options out there. Team sports teach kids about working together for a common goal, and exposes them to the challenges of competition. These are both excellent skills that your child will need when he or she grows up and has to cope with the real world. Granted, we've all heard the horror stories of parents or coaches who get too caught up in the drive to win and overlook the children's needs—this sort of thing is never good for the kids. However, I truly believe that a low-key competitive edge, coupled with an education in the principles of cooperation and good sportsmanship, will help children become high-achievers when they become adults.

Finding the right team for your child may take a little searching. You want to match your child's interests and abilities with any sports program because participation should, above all, be *fun*. Contact your local Parks and Recreation Department or get in touch with your community's Civic Center or Chamber of Commerce—these organizations often maintain lists of locally sponsored teams. And, before you sign your child up, make a point of attending a game or two and talk to the coaches, organizers, and other parents. Does every kid get a chance to play, or is the field monopolized by one or two "stars"? Does the coach seem to be sensitive to the different ability-levels of his team members? These kinds of observations will give you a sense of the team's priorities. Your goal is to find a team that puts the children's enjoyment and skill development over playing to win.

COMPONENTS OF FITNESS

In my practice, I'm often called upon to give lectures to community organizations about the importance of fitness—for kids *and* for adults. One thing everybody seems to be curious about is how different types of exercise offer different physical benefits. In today's society, where everything is "niche-marketed" and specialized, it seems like there's a lot of different, "specialty" exercise programs, with new ones popping up every day. But don't let all of those ads confuse you.

There are really only 5 components of physical fitness—those "specialty" programs simply focus on just one or a couple of them. However, a well-rounded fitness regimen would include some exercises that are aimed at each of the components, which are:

- flexibility
- muscular strength
- muscular endurance
- cardiovascular or aerobic conditioning
- body composition

Let's take a closer look at each one and examine what they're designed to do.

Flexibility

Flexibility is the ability of each muscle group and joint to work through it's full range of movement. This entails a lot of stretching, which is essential to keep the body limber and prevent injury, like muscle strains. The benefits? Better balance and better posture are two, but flexibility exercises are also important for good joint mobility and for limbering up the muscles and tendons. This is why stretching or warming up is always recommended before more strenuous exercise.

But stretching isn't just for limbering up and preventing injury during exercise—it's important in everything we do, every day. Think of how often you have to reach up over your head to get something on a high shelf, or bend down to pick up something you've dropped. That involves stretching—and without flexibility, even these everyday actions can become difficult, painful or even downright impossible!

Muscular Strength.

Muscular strength is the force a muscle can exert to accomplish an action. Exercises geared to developing strength put your muscles to the test, challenging you to use your muscles to their utmost ability. For example, you would lift weights that are almost (but not quite) the heaviest that you can lift. If you're on an exercise bike, you set the controls to increase the resistance of the pedals, making them harder to pump. You're always pushing yourself to the outer limit of your current ability.

But children should not be involved in strength training on their own—and neither should adults, for that matter! You should always get instruction from a qualified fitness professional first. And it's really not a good idea for kids to be involved in a strength training program, anyway. Their bodies are still developing and are therefore very vulnerable to injury. Opt, instead to involve them in the next component: muscular endurance.

Muscular Endurance

Endurance is how long or how often a muscle can exert a force—like carrying a weight or repeating an activity—without becoming fatigued. Like strength training, this type of exercise also pits your muscles against resistance, but at a lower level. The benefits here are found in the repetition of the exercise, or in holding a particular position (muscular contraction) for a certain period of time. Working with light weights, doing push-ups, pull-ups, or sit-ups, and calisthenics like leg lifts are all muscular endurance activities.

Many experts agree that kids should not start out building endurance by using weights. They need to learn to control their form and technique first, or else they risk injury. Once they've mastered the technique of an exercise and have developed adequate muscle control, they can use elastic exercise bands or even 16 ounce vegetable cans as home-made one-pound weights. But equipment isn't always needed. Even pumping your legs to make a swing go higher builds endurance! Just keep in mind that it's easy for anybody, not just kids, to injure themselves if they don't maintain proper form and control. That's why this sort of activity becomes risky when kids are tired or distracted.

Cardiovascular or Aerobic

Aerobic means "with oxygen"—this type of exercise is designed to strengthen the heart and speed up it's delivery of oxygen to your muscles by increasing the flow of blood, which carries the oxygen. It's for this reason that aerobic activity is also known as cardiovascular or cardiorespiratory exercise. It involves strenuously exercising the large muscle groups (such as the quadriceps, hamstrings, and gluteal muscles in the lower body; or the biceps, triceps, latissimus dorsi, trapezius, and pectorals in the upper body). All of this forces the heart to increase it's delivery of blood —and oxygen—to the muscles that are being worked. In other words, you're not only giving your arms and legs a workout, your also putting your heart and lungs, and your circulatory and respiratory systems, through their paces. Good examples would be rollerblading, skating, swimming, jogging and bike riding for periods of 30 minutes or longer.

Body Composition

This last component of exercise isn't an exercise at all. Instead, body composition refers to the ratio of lean body mass to fat.

Lean body mass includes your muscles, organs, bones, skin, blood, and nervous system; whereas fat is the stored adipose tissue that insulates the organs and basically just sits there until it's needed to be burned as a source of energy. One of the key benefits of any exercise program is its ability to optimize body composition—the ratio of lean body mass to fat.

KIDS HAVE SPECIAL NEEDS

All of the exercise components described above offer great benefits, but there are some special issues to consider when it comes to our children. Remember, kids are not just little adults —their bodies are very different—they're forever growing and constantly changing. You have to make sure that any program you involve them in doesn't put too much strain on their systems. For example, if your child is involved in aerobics, it's very important to make sure that there's a cool-down period afterwards. This is because during the activity, the blood flow to the exercising muscles is increased and stopping abruptly can lead to blood pooling and fainting.

Similarly, it's important to know that strength-training programs carry certain risks for kids. Heavy stress placed on still-developing bones and muscles can distort bone and ligament development, especially during growth-spurt periods, and improper form can lead to injury. That's why many experts discourage strength training for children under the age of 12—they're usually not physically disciplined enough to avoid hurting themselves! But if your child is adamant about participating in some form of strength-training, perhaps to be like an older sibling, family member or sports idol, then at least make sure he or she is properly supervised, and that the progression is *very slow*. There's a "10 percent" rule for adults, which says that you should never increase the weight, duration, or intensity of an exercise by more than 10 percent at a time—and kids should progress even more slowly than *that!* In addition, it's important to include flexibility exercises, before and after the session, to insure that the surrounding tendons, joints, and ligaments are supple enough to withstand the stress.

According to the American Academy of Pediatrics (AAP), low-stress endurance-training exercises can be a good thing for kids, but once again, supervision and proper instruction is paramount. When properly done, endurance training has a positive effect on muscle tone, fosters positive changes in musculature development, and helps children feel good about themselves and their abilities.

My personal recommendation? For kids 12 and under, I suggest that you start simply—with fun, gentle activities, pacing the child's progress according to his or her developing abilities. For example, young children really can't lift their own body weight initially, so you might want to take them to the park to go climbing or try out the monkey bars and swings. Who needs to lift weights when there are trees to climb, rocks to pile up into a fort and other fun things to do?!

A NOTE ABOUT DEHYDRATION

Whatever approach to exercise and physical activity you choose for your child—even if they're just out playing in the yard—it's important that you be aware of the risk of dehydration and work to prevent it. Young children (those who have not yet reached puberty) are much more vulnerable to heat stress and dehydration than adolescents and adults. That's because young children produce more heat during an activity than adults—they have a larger ratio of surface area to body mass. And they are less efficient getting rid of the heat—children's sweat glands put out less than half that of adults.

When kids are outside in the heat—especially when the temperature reaches 80 degrees or more—or in humid conditions, they need to be encouraged to drink lots of water, cut down on the time they spend outside, and even tone down the intensity of their running around. And as a parent, you should be alert to the tell-tale signs of heat exhaustion. These are:

- redness of the cheeks

- profuse sweating

- lightheaded or dizziness

- nausea

- clammy skin

- rapid but weak pulse or heart beat

- chills

- shortness of breath

- lack of saliva

- pasty-looking tongue

If you see these signs, get the children out of the heat and into an air-conditioned room or at least a shady area, and give them plenty of fluids: 4 to 8 ounces every 15 minutes. It's best to stick with water—sugary sodas or fruit drinks are harder to digest and can cause stomach upset.

If heat exhaustion is left unattended it can become heat stroke. Symptoms include:

- dry, hot skin

- lack of sweat

- very rapid pulse

- dizziness

- loss of balance

- headache

- flushed skin

In severe cases of heat stroke, shock and unconsciousness can occur. If this happens, put your child into cold water, hold him under a cold shower, or hold ice to the back of his neck and get medical attention *immediately*! This is a life-threatening situation. If your child has already become unconscious or seems to be in shock, elevate his feet.

Even garden-variety dehydration, long before it turns into heat exhaustion or heat stroke, is dangerous. When a person is dehydrated, the heart rate, blood pressure, and body temperature increases, while the flow of blood to the skin decreases. Our body relies on perspiration to maintain body temperature—sweat on the skin helps to cool the body down as it dries. But with perspiration comes a loss of body fluids—the fluids our organs need to function efficiently.

Young children are at special risk from over-exertion and dehydration. They sweat less and are inclined to push themselves to their extreme limits during play, so their bodies can overheat much more easily than adults and teenagers. This means that they'll become dehydrated much more quickly than their older siblings or their parents. That's why I recommend that anyone supervising a child in an exercise program should keep the pace light at first, and make certain that there are plenty of water breaks. And as I said earlier, plain water is fine. Sometimes kids are more willing to drink diluted fruit juice, and if that's true for you, I recommend 2 ounces of real fruit juice to 6 ounces of water. Skip the sports drinks unless your child is exercising rigorously for more than an hour or two—and even then they *don't* need a 20 ounce bottle in a single serving! In hot, humid climates or during the summer months in more temperate areas, you need to be especially vigilant about water breaks and rest periods.

In addition, your child's individual physical characteristics can make a difference in how susceptible he or she might be to becoming dehydrated. Dehydration strikes more quickly in children who are larger in size or who have a higher percentage of body fat. In addition, boys are more susceptible than girls because they tend to sweat more. The clothing a child wears can also make a difference in their ability to sweat and maintain their body temperature. The best clothing is loose, light-weight, and 100 percent cotton— cotton "breathes" easier.

Above all, make sure that the kids drink fluids before, during, and after any exercise. Carbonated and caffeine-based drinks are much less effective than water or diluted fruit juice. In fact, caffeinated drinks can actually make the problem worse, because caffine is a diuretic, so it actually speeds up the loss of body fluid instead of helping replace the fluids that have been lost. Get kids into the habit of drinking at least 8 ounces of water before any strenuous activity, then at least 4 ounces every 15 minutes. After the activity is over they should get another 8 ounces—and don't wait for them to tell you they're thirsty! By the time they actually feel thirsty, their body is already at a loss for fluid!

MAKING IT ALL WORK (OUT)

By now you're probably convinced that exercise is important but, if you're like many over-worked parents, you may feel there just aren't enough hours in the day to make time for your kids to play. Well, there really *are* ways to solve the problem—it just takes a little creativity to come up with solutions. In Chapters 12 and 13 we'll go into a lot of fitness-related activities you can get your family involved in, and we'll provide solutions to lots of common problems parents have in developing a fitness program for their kids. For now, however, start looking around at the resources available in your area. If time's a problem and your child is still fairly young, talk to a few other parents about setting up a play group and take turns hosting one—sort of like car-pooling or play dates—only these play dates have a purpose!

If your child is interested in participating in a structured sport, you can use the same "time-sharing" principle with the parents of other children on the team. You can take turns being the one to drive the kids to the event and cheer them on. And while you're there, *pay attention!* There's nothing more disheartening to a child than trying to get his parents' attention when he's out on the field, only to see they're busily talking on their cell-phone. To be honest with you, that's worse than not being there at all.

I should warn you, however, that "time-sharing" attendance with other parents is not the most satisfying solution—at least, not from your child's perspective. A parent's attendance is very important to children, and believe me, they will be disappointed if you're not there to watch. I know this is the case with Alexander, so I've decided to make a few sacrifices to be there for him, no matter how inconvenient it may be. And I'm convinced that this has paid off. Being there for the events has contributed to the strong bond we share between us.

And, looking beyond the organized activities, remember that the best thing you can do is just get out there and play with your kids. Toss a ball around with them. Get active. The kids don't care if you're a great athlete—they just want to have fun and share some time with you. If time is tight, don't worry. You don't have to do 30 minutes or an hour all at once—15 minute spurts are just fine. Just make sure it's an *active* 15 minutes. How to tell? Try the "talk test": if you can sing, you're not working hard enough, but if you can't talk, you're working too hard.

Above all, have fun. That's the point, after all: teaching your kids to recognize that using their bodies is pleasurable, and showing them that it's something they should continue to do throughout their entire lives!

NUTRITION THRU THE AGES

7

$\mathcal{A}$ child's growth and development can be divided into 4 stages, which are based on their growth rate and activity level. Though I am defining them in specific years within this text, it is important to recognize that there is some overlap between the stages. Remember: children grow at their own rate and some may enter into a particular category before—or after—their actual age.

We begin with infancy, which starts at birth and ends when a child turns a year old. During infancy there is a major growth spurt accompanied by many physiological changes—all of which result in increased nutritional demands. Next come the early childhood years, from about age 1 through 5. During this time, the rate of growth slows down somewhat and maintains a more steady pace, but nutritional needs are still high, as young children tend to be very physically active.

School age children, aged 6 through about 10, are on the threshold of another period of rapid growth, which introduces a new set of nutritional demands. Finally, adolescence, from the ages of approximately 11 to 18, is another time of growth spurts, accompanied by major bodily changes.

Because each stage and every child is different, nutrition can't be "one size fits all." Instead, you have to tailor your plans to suit the specific needs of your own child, based on his or her current stage of development, and you have to be ready to alter this program as your child's needs change. This really isn't hard to do once you have a good understanding of how children's needs change over time. That's exactly what I'm hoping you'll learn in this chapter. The essential nutrients that we discussed in the previous chapter are important throughout your child's life, but the amounts required will vary significantly at each stage of development. Let's take a look at each of these developmental stages more closely, so that you can get a better picture of the nutrients required at every age and stage of your child's life.

SOME GENERAL OBSERVATIONS ABOUT BOYS AND GIRLS

During infancy and early childhood, boys are usually taller and heavier than girls. During pre-adolescence, however, the opposite is true, as girls tend to hit puberty a couple of years before boys do. Girls reach puberty—and start a period accompanied by rapid growth and hormonal changes—somewhere between age 9 and 13. Boys, on the other hand, typically begin their road to puberty at about 13. This size difference continues in the girls' favor for awhile, but eventually the boys catch up and move ahead. Girls tend to reach their adult height by age 17, whereas boys continue to get taller until they're about 21.

And there's also a difference in the *kind* of weight they gain. During childhood, boys and girls gain about the same amount of lean body mass (muscle and bone), but girls have a higher proportion of body fat. After age 13, boys experience a rapid increase in lean body mass that continues until late adolescence. Girls, on the other hand, usually attain their peak lean body mass by age 15. The end result is that males wind up with about 12 percent body fat, while girls develop twice that amount, or 24 percent.

Boys and girls also grow up with very different sets of expectations, due to the gender-based biases of family, friends, and society in general. The culture projects an ideal of waify thinness for females, and mega-muscularity for boys and men (just think of all those TV ads for "six-pack abs," not to mention the muscle-bound heroes and villains portrayed on TV and video games).

Parents also tend to impose gender-based biases of their own. Many, and quite possibly most, parents tend to treat girls as more fragile than boys. Boys are expected to be strong, both physically and emotionally, while girls are expected to be nurturing and passive. So parents are more likely to encourage their sons to get actively involved in strenuous play but much less likely to do so with their daughters. And, unfortunately, daughters are much more likely to be encouraged to "watch what they eat" if they seem larger than their peers, while boys are simply described as being of "husky" build.

Unlike the differences in physiological development, the cultural differences between boys and girls are largely the result of expectations. Want proof? Look at households where there are siblings of both sexes. Girls in a household of brothers often become "tom boyish"—the result of being exposed to and included in their brothers games. (Although sometimes they go to the other extreme, being more protected and emotional, if they're treated as the "little porcelain doll" in the family.) Similarly, boys who are raised with lots of sisters often end up being included in so-called "girls games" and frequently end up displaying some of the same sensitivity and nurturing traits that their siblings do.

The thing to note is that most of these differences aren't apparent early on. During infancy and toddlerhood, boys and girls seem to be interested in much the same things and play in much the same way. It's only as they approach preschool that differences begin to appear, which suggests that it is environmental change—the influence of cultural expectations, the desire to fit in with other kids, the opportunities that they are provided—that causes the sudden development of stereo-typically "male" and "female" behaviors.

CALCULATING CHANGING PROTEIN REQUIREMENTS

One thing many people find difficult to understand is how protein needs change as a child grows. In fact, calculating a person's actual protein requirement, no matter what stage of life he or she has reached, is pretty simple. Say your child weighs 42 pounds at age four. Just multiply that number by .55 grams and you've got the recommended daily protein intake. Similarly, if your 8-year-old weighs 78 pounds, multiply that by .6 grams and you've got a good idea of how much protein he or she should be getting.

Baby Steps: Birth to 1 Year

Under normal conditions, infants and toddlers need 4 to 5 cups of fluid each day to meet their basic requirement for water. Of course, that volume can change when conditions are less than ideal. For example, if a child is ill with a fever or is suffering from vomiting and diarrhea, fluid needs will increase. With a child this young, you can't use thirst to indicate fluid needs—in fact, thirst is a bad indicator of fluid needs at any age because by the time you feel thirsty, your body's already past the point of needing rehydrating! But there *are* a few clues to look for. For example, if you notice that you're changing fewer wet diapers, or that your child's urine is dark in color or has a strong ammonia-like odor, you're probably seeing the early warning signs of dehydration. Other signs include nausea, clammy skin, and a "fuzzy" or coated tongue.

Food Needs

When it comes to meeting your infant's nutritional needs, you need to know that babies need relatively more iron, calcium, and zinc in the early stages of life than at any other time, because they're in a period of very rapid growth.

Breast milk is the ideal food for this first year of life, because it provides the necessary quantity of all the nutrients. I realize, however, that breast feeding is not for everyone, and if you choose to go with bottle feeding, there are nutritionally sound alternatives available to you. Cow's milk is not recommended for babies under a year old because it's hard for them to digest and because it lacks iron, but iron-fortified formulas are fine. Iron-fortified soy-based formulas are a good choice if you suspect your infant might have an allergy to the dairy based variety.

Breast milk or fortified formula is all your baby needs for the first six months of life. Once the child weighs at least 13 pounds, can sit with support, and opens his or her mouth in anticipation of an approaching spoonful of food, you can start introducing solids into the diet. Breast-feeding Moms can start offering a bottle, at this stage, too, (if they so choose). But don't rush the process—introducing solid foods too early can increase the risk of food allergies.

Making Changes as You Go. . .

Once a baby turns one year old, it's fine to start giving whole milk—but DO NOT give skim, no-fat, or low-fat milk or dairy products to a child of this age. In fact, low-fat or skim milk should never be offered to children under the age of 2 because they need the fat in their diet to foster the development of their nervous system, brain and cognitive function. To be honest with you, I recommend you refrain from giving processed "fat-free" products to growing children of any age!

What sort of solids should you introduce? I suggest you keep it simple and basic: a rice-based cereal—especially if it's iron-fortified—is a safe choice, and it's a good idea to use apple juice instead of water to mix the cereal. The vitamin C in the apple juice will help the your baby's body to absorb the iron (but don't use orange juice for this because it's too acidic for a very young child's tummy). Then, gradually, as your child shows a willingness to try new things, begin to introduce other new foods, one at a time.

The reason for this one-at-a-time approach is simple—it's the best way to avoid food allergy problems. If you introduce a new food, then wait a couple of days before introducing another, you have a better chance of pinpointing the offending food if an allergy occurs. Stick with pureed veggies at first, then fruits, but avoid wheat, eggs, cow's milk, peanut butter and strawberries, because these foods frequently trigger allergic reactions in very young children. And *never* add honey or corn syrup to foods at this age, because they can carry organisms that cause botulism—and babies' digestive systems are extremely vulnerable to such bacteria-borne ailments.

Infants eat often—usually every 2 to 4 hours, and the average feeding will consist of 6 to 8 ounces of milk or formula. A steady weight gain is your indicator that your infant is eating enough—after the first week of life, an average infant will gain about 7 ounces per week during the first 3 months, and by 6 months of age will have approximately doubled his or her birth weight. After that, the pace of growth generally slows down a bit, with the weekly weight gain dropping to about 2 to 3 ounces.

As long as your child is staying more or less on track with weight gain, don't force feeding times. Some parents offer a bottle every time a child cries, but this is not a good practice to get into, because babies cry for many reasons, not just from hunger. Others add cereal to "bulk-up" the formula, hoping that it will get the baby to sleep longer through the night, but all this does is put the child into a "food coma" (sort of like the groggy way adults feel after eating too much Thanksgiving turkey!).

Overfeeding like this is never a good idea—after all, healthful eating habits start in infancy! What's more, overfeeding during early childhood often leads to obesity later on. Why? Because it teaches infants to ignore their body's signals of satiety (fullness), and conditions them to eat whenever food is available. Even in infants, when the body takes in more food than it needs, it stores the excess calories as fat, and if babies are continually over-fed, their bodies will begin to manufacture more fat-storage cells. Extra storage cells created in infancy can mean a lifetime of struggles with weight for your child later in life!

EXPLORING THE WORLD: AGES 2 TO 5

During the pre-school years, the early rapid growth and development rate begins to slow down. However, toddlers and pre-schoolers are *very* active, when they're allowed to be—and this increased activity means new nutritional needs. To put this in terms of the Food Pyramid, here's a basic breakdown:

Recommended Daily Servings, by Food Group		
	Age 2 to 4	*Age 5 (and 6)*
Milk/Dairy	3-5 svgs (4 oz each)	3 svgs (8 oz each)
Meat	2 svgs (2 oz each)	3-4 svgs (2 oz each)
Fruits/Veggies	All age groups: at least 5 colorful servings	
Grains	All age groups: 6 to 12 servings	
Fats/oils	3 tsps/day	3 Tbsp/day

For young kids a fruit or vegetable serving is 1 tablespoon for every year they are old. So a 3 year old's applesauce serving would be 3 tablespoons. For older kids—between 5 and 6 years old—a serving is 1 medium fruit, or 1/2 cup cooked veggies or fruit, or 1 cup raw veggies.

For younger kids a serving of grains is 1/2 slice of bread or a tablespoon of grain or cereal for every year of their age. For older kids it's a whole slice of bread, 1/2 cup noodles, potatoes, or cereal, or 1/3 cup rice or legumes.

When it comes to fats and oils, it's beneficial to remember, they're also getting fat that is innately found in animal protein, dairy foods, nuts and grains. And these servings are just guides. A child's appetite will vary each day so if they're hungrier, by all means let their hunger level guide you.

After age 2, the milk servings can be skim or 2-percent milk, as long as there's enough calories in the diet from other sources. But remember, before age 2, only whole milk should be used. And also keep in mind that these suggested servings are only averages— your child's actual needs will depend upon body size, growth rate and activity levels, among other factors.

It's easy to understand why protein is so important during this age group. Young children are inherently very active and growing steadily, so they need adequate protein for healthy development. But remember that protein is not stored in the body —excess protein is converted to glucose for use as energy. And protein makes very *expensive* glucose! It's also important to remember that, while there are similarities that stretch across this entire age range, there are differences in nutritional and fitness needs across the Early Childhood stage itself. Let's take a closer look.

The "Terrible" 1s and 2s

Young toddlers have entered the wonderful world of solid foods. They've begun to acquire a few teeth and have learned to bite through a variety of textures. If you start off with soft or soft-cooked, chopped table foods, you can expand their food horizons while making them a part of the whole family-dinner experience. Just be sure to avoid foods that can cause choking: nuts, hot dogs, raw apple or carrots, whole grapes, and hard candy! I like to use the "dime rule." A young child's esophagus is about the size of a dime, so you want to avoid giving any foods that tiny because they could get lodged in the throat and choke them.

But most toddlers are notoriously picky eaters. There's even a name for it: *food neophobia* or a fear of trying new foods. Of course, you can be a food neophobe at any age, but it's extremely common in kids. Still, it's important to realize that children's taste preferences are not set in stone—they can be altered by exposure to new foods, as long as you're very patient and gentle about introducing them.

Parents who overcompensate for neophobia by coercing kids into eating, or by caving in to their demands and giving them only what they choose for themselves, are setting themselves up for mealtime problems for as long as the child lives at home! When dinnertime is confrontational, kids will just dig in their heels and increase their resistence. If you end up playing everybody's personal chef, making different meals for everybody in the family, you're just encouraging finicky eating. Instead, remember that children will generally eat what the family eats, if there's no other option, and if you serve at least one familiar food that they like with each meal, you can be sure they'll eat something.

The key to introducing new foods is patience. It may take a number of exposures—maybe 10, 15, or even 20—before a child will voluntary accept a new food, but persistence will pay off. And by age 2, kids will establish eating patterns that can remain with them throughout life. So it's best to encourage a little adventure: offer toddlers a variety of foods—and the same foods prepared in a variety of ways—to allow them to explore and discover their own likes and dislikes.

But despite your best efforts to encourage variety, your kids will probably still go through "food jags"—stages where they only like a certain small handful of foods and refuse to eat anything else. Most children go through quite a few food jags while growing up. But these temporary bouts are nothing to worry about. Your child is probably eating more than you realize, and if you're making sure that he or she is getting the necessary nutrients by offering healthful foods, things will be just fine in the long run.

Here are a few strategies you can try to overcome food neophobias and food jags:

- Try not to make an issue of a sudden food jag. It will only inspire your child to resist you even harder, which will only delay the return to normal eating patterns.

- Serve food in small portions and use colorful, kid-sized bowls, plates, utensils and cups. It's less intimidating than food served on adult-sized plates—and more fun.

- Make the presentation of the food colorful and fun—visual stimulation is important and can tempt children to try something they'd otherwise reject.

If you need ideas for some age-appropriate, tempting dishes check out Chapter 11 for some sample meals.

Feeding Frenzy

When it comes to feeding toddlers, mealtime can be downright frustrating! Once you realize why they act as they do, it'll be easier to deal with the situation. For example, parents are often mystified by an abrupt decrease in appetite but this commonly occurs when a child approaches the age of 2. This is a normal process, because it's the time when the extremely rapid growth rate of infancy begins to slow down. This means that a child's overall need for calories is also lower. Don't worry—as the child becomes more and more active, his or her appetite will increase again.

The most important point I want to emphasize is this: *NEVER* force your child to eat. Forget the old-fashioned rule that children can't leave the table unless they clean their plate. Over the years, researchers have found that it's better to let young children eat when they are hungry and stop when they are satisfied—*NOT* full. Besides, small children have smaller stomachs than adults do, so they tend to become satiated faster. They're also more likely to become hungry faster. Thus, it's probably best to allow a small child to eat 5 or 6 small, mini-meals daily, instead of sitting down to 2 or 3 larger ones—but make sure that at least 2 of these mini-meals coincide with regular family mealtimes, for family mealtimes are very important at every age.

From 2 to 5

All kids grow at their own rate. If you took a handful of healthy 5 year olds and compared their sizes and shapes, they could range from 3 to 4-1/2 feet tall and weigh anywhere from 35 to 80 pounds. And if you followed their growth over the course of a year, you'd see that their growing patterns will vary from one child to the next. You can't just go with a number on the bathroom scale—and with really young children the Body Mass Index (BMI) isn't always accurate either. But if your child is gaining about 5 to 6 pounds per year at this stage, and if they're adding about 2 inches in height, they're probably on the right track.

The good thing is that as pre-schoolers grow in size and strength, they're also growing in awareness and acquiring greater communication skills. It's an opportune time to teach your children about healthy foods and explain why they're important to their body. And at this stage you can even enlist them in helping you with your efforts to design a healthy lifestyle for the family!

For example, young children can help you prepare meals. They are quite capable of helping to set the table, mix foods, and even put certain foods out on plates. You can also begin working with their food likes and dislikes cooperatively. If a child doesn't want to try something, you can establish a one-bite policy: "Try one bite and then you can leave the rest." This gets them to take a taste without feeling forced to eat it all—sometimes they're pleasantly surprised, and the new food can even become a favorite!

SCHOOL AGERS: 6 TO 10 YEARS OLD

When kids reach school age, they've got a whole new world to conquer. But while they're out conquering the playground and the classroom, they're also moving away from the time when their parents were the biggest influence in their lives. With this new world comes new influences—some good, some not so good. They also spend a big chunk of their days away from home and away from your ability to keep a watchful eye out for their well-being.

As they begin to master formal educational skills, they face new challenges and demands, and embark on a whole new aspect of their development. Just as their physical development demands proper nutrition, so does their intellectual development. A healthy diet is crucial now, not only to provide the energy they need to grow and be active, but to sharpen their senses and their minds.

New Changes and Pressures

Once children start school, many factors affect the quality and quantity of their food intake. First of all, parents suddenly find that they have less control over what their kids are eating. For the first time at least one meal (usually lunch but sometimes breakfast or a snack, too) is regularly eaten away from home. Unfortunately, even if you pack your children lunch, you can't be sure they're eating all those good, healthy choices—they could just as easily be trading that banana for a friend's cupcake or donut. And lots of schools actively encourage the purchase of not-so-healthy fast- food from the kiosks in the cafeteria, and junk foods from vending machines installed on school grounds—innovations that have been justified by some schools as a source of revenues to beef up the school budget.

After school, kids are also likely to begin spending some time away from home, perhaps visiting at a friend's house or participating in an after care program, and once again you have little opportunity to oversee the kinds of snacks or junk food they're getting into. The result? Your kids' eating schedules are likely to become erratic—and their nutrition may very well suffer for it.

A Difficult Contradiction

Kids have a hard time maintaining healthy eating habits during their school years. Just as parents no longer have complete control over their children's nutrition once they're off to school, children also lose some of the control they're used to— they suddenly can't eat when they're hungry because they're stuck following the school's rigid schedule. It's just one more factor that breaks down the child's ability to tune into his or her own body's cues. And yet studies consistently show that good nutrition is crucial to top performance in school. Not only do hungry children have difficulty concentrating in class, but a healthy diet is vital to fuel the steady growth they're experiencing during this stage. "School agers" (actually beginning at the age of 5) typically average a growth rate of about 7 pounds and 2 inches per year!

This stage is also a critical point for parents because it's your best opportunity to prevent weight problems before they occur. If, on the other hand, a child becomes overweight during their early school years, chances are he or she will be stuck fighting a weight problem for the rest of their life. Rapid weight gain during this stage means an increase in the size and number of fat storage cells—and these cells never go away. The more you develop, the greater the tendency of the body to retain weight.

And by the way, watch out for a common mistake made by many parents—treating sons differently from daughters at meal times. Too often parents overlook it when boys eat large portions, but they start obsessing if a daughter does the same. This is detrimental for both the boys and the girls. Boys who eat to excess are just as likely as girls to become overweight—and calling them "chunky" or "husky" doesn't reduce the very real health risks that go along with obesity. At the same time, parental obsession over a daughter's weight at an early age will cause her to develop negative and debilitating attitudes about her body image and most likely ruin her self esteem. Remember: You are still the most influential person in your child's life and disapproval from you during these vulnerable years can be devastating!

The Pre-Teen Years: Ages 7 to 12

The pre-teen years are a transitional stage. It's a time when the body prepares to shift from the slow, steady growth of the school-age child into the major growth spurt of puberty and adolescence. Some children, particularly girls, actually begin puberty during this early stage, while others will show no signs of puberty until a few more years have passed. That means you'll want to be particularly aware of where your child is along the spectrum and determine their changing needs during this transitional period.

First of all, they'll be needing more of certain nutrients than they used to—protein, calcium, and iron, in particular. Iron is especially important for girls who begin menstruating early. Second, the food guide pyramid will be similar to the 6 and under for the less mature, and more like the puberty period for the more mature.

Puberty and Adolescence: Ages 11 to 18

During adolescence kids attain 15 to 25 percent of their adult height and they nearly double their weight. This is a period of irregular growth spurts and a time when boys and girls will both experience a great deal of anxiety about their bodies. Many unfamiliar hormonal and physical changes are occurring quite rapidly and at the same time. Boys have to deal with vocal changes, girls deal with the onset of menstruation, and both deal with the sudden appearance of pimples. Girls worry about the changes in their body proportion and boys feel awkward as their growth spurts cause them to shoot up in height before their weight has a chance to catch up. Both boys *and* girls are either worried that they're not developing fast enough, or that they're developing too fast. And all of this is happening at a time when boys and girls, having newly discovered the attraction of the opposite sex, are busy trying to impress each other.

Keeping Up With Changing Food Needs

To accommodate for all of the new physical changes that pubescent and adolescent bodies are going through, their nutritional requirements change once again. Here's how the Food Guide Pyramid would look for puberty and beyond:

11 to 18 Years Old	
Milk/Dairy	3-5 svgs (8 oz)
Meat	3-4 svgs (2-4 oz)
Fruit/Vegetables	at least 5 colorful servings from these groups (preferably 8-10)
Grains	8 to 12 servings is ideal, with at least 6 coming from whole grains
Fats/Oils	3 Tbsp

Note that the biggest change here is in the protein group—which makes sense given how much growing is going on during this time. Calcium needs also increase, to accommodate this final stage of skeletal growth, and 1,200 to 1,500 milligrams daily is the recommended amount. Iron needs are also high at this time—a daily average of 8 to 18 milligrams is recommended. There's an increased need for iron in both boys *and* girls. Boys need it for the intense period of muscle growth they're going through, but in the teen years, girls needs are higher, because of the blood lost each month during menstruation (they need the iron to make more blood).

Amazing Growth

During adolescence, body weight in both boys and girls increases dramatically. Boys gain an average of 57 pounds during this time, and girls generally gain about 45 pounds. In boys, most of this new weight goes to muscle, but a girl's body is beginning to prepare itself for childbearing, by producing higher levels of estrogen, which naturally promotes the accumulation of body fat.

At the same time, the skeleton is growing rapidly, too. During the teen years, bone acquires 50 percent of its lifetime growth—no wonder there's such a large need for calcium. In fact, the *overall* nutritional needs of adolescents are higher than they would be for an adult of the same size and probably higher than they'll be during any other stage of their life, precisely because they're bodies are undergoing such intense growth. Parents of teenage boys will testify to this—boys during adolescence will eat you out of house and home!

The problem is, all of this growth may trigger some pretty high levels of stress in adolescents and teens. Their bodily changes may make them feel self-conscious and uncomfortable. This is precisely why dieting and eating disorders are so common during the teen years. We'll explore these problems in detail in the next few chapters, but right now it's important to understand that there are some steps you can take to help alleviate feelings of inadequacy from developing into anything more serious than an awkward phase. And the most important step of all is simple, open and non-judgmental communication.

Much of the stress and anxiety that teens experience occurs because they don't really understand what's happening to their bodies. You can help them immensely by talking to them about this well in advance. In fact, it's not a bad idea to begin discussions about puberty and "the birds and the bees" as early as 7 or 8 years old. It's better that they learn the truth from you instead of the fallacies they're likely to get from their overly imaginative schoolmates.

Let them know about the changes they will experience during puberty ahead of time. Explain that it's a normal part of growing up, and reassure them that all of their friends will eventually go through it too. They also need to know that this stage is temporary and will someday end. This reassurance won't remove *all of* the stress of adolescence, of course—it goes with the territory—but it *will* help.

Part Three

Dealing With Dysfunctional Eating

IF YOUR CHILD
IS OVERWEIGHT

8

$\mathcal{I}$ see it all the time in my practice: parents worrying about their child's weight, wondering if he or she should be put on a diet—and the poor kid is only 5, 6, or 7 years old! Sure, the child may be slightly heavier than other kids of the same age, but when I ask a few questions, I usually discover that the excess weight is predominantly because the child simply isn't *doing* anything. No exercise. No healthy running around in the back yard. Nothing!

This is not to say that the children of American aren't collectively facing a real problem with regard to weight. Childhood obesity, like its adult counterpart, is becoming a national epidemic! It's just that if a child is slightly chubby, it rarely poses real health concerns—certainly not enough to justify medication or the emotional turmoil that goes with putting the child on a diet. The best solution for overweight children is to make certain that there's enough healthy activity in their day, and that they're getting adequate nutrition for their age and physical needs.

In fact, good nutrition and healthy, vigorous activity is almost always the best way to go, even for children who are more than just "a little chubby." Diets are almost never an appropriate first choice for treatment (as you'll learn in the next chapter). But while this is true, even for cases of true childhood obesity, I believe that there are other things that you may need to do as well—things that will help to strengthen your child's sense of self-esteem and assure him or

129

her of your unconditional love and support. Why? Because in addition to the physical costs of childhood obesity—both as a cause of illness during childhood and as the main controllable factor associated with disease later in life—there are mental and emotional costs too. And those costs can be debilitating, leaving a scar for life.

OBESITY VERSUS OVERWEIGHT

First of all, it's important to distinguish between being slightly "husky," truly overweight, and obese. Here's how the Centers for Disease Control distinguish the terms. They call a person "overweight" when body weight is greater than the norm for height. "Obesity," on the other hand, specifically refers to fat: it means that the ratio of body fat to lean muscle mass is greater than normal—this usually translates into a body weight that is 20 percent or more above the norm for height. In other words, obesity means having too much fat, whereas a person who is overweight may not have much fat at all. That's because lean body mass— muscle tissue—weighs more than fat, and a highly muscular person can easily weigh more than normal for his height.

So how do you tell if your child's weight is likely to cause problems? One "unscientific" way is to check the size of clothes they're wearing, right? You know what I mean—"She used to be a Junior size 5, but now she wears a size 9." Well, those size numbers are pretty much meaningless, these days. Why? Because clothing manufacturers will use any ploy to guarantee sales of their products —including vanity. They know that people want to believe that they're wearing smaller sizes, so they've changed the way they label their clothes. As the rate of obesity has climbed, the sizes on the labels of clothing have changed, especially with the Junior and Women sizes, so that a Junior size 5 today is actually bigger than the size 5s of a decade ago!

Men's clothing is less misleading—they're traditionally based on specific measurements (waist size, inseam length, and so forth). But when it comes to women's and girls' clothing—and clothes for preschool boys, too—that number on the size tag says nothing meaningful for you to rely upon.

On a more "scientific" front, there are charts and tables that try to tell us what people should weigh. A couple of decades ago, health professionals were using the old "height and weight" charts that were developed by the Metropolitan Life Insurance Company in 1959. They're what you probably remember from when *you* were a kid—the charts that established an 'ideal weight' for various heights based on whether a person was small, medium. or large framed (whatever *that* meant). According to these old charts, the weight range for a 5'5" woman extended from a mere 117 pounds (for a small frame) to 150 pounds (for a large frame).

What's wrong with those old charts? A couple of things. First of all, the "frame" categories were pretty vague. Second of all, they didn't distinguish between fat weight and muscle weight. Also, remember the source that was used to come up with the data. Met Life is an insurance company, and it developed its weight categories from the data on the insurance policy forms of its claimants—people who had died. These people are *not* true representatives of the general population. The information was distorted, over-representing people with some pretty serious physical problems: malnourished alcoholics, smokers, and the like. So the "normal" weights tended to be set very low.

To overcome these problems, in 1988 a researcher developed a new way to calculate weight, using a chart called the Body Mass Index, or BMI. Its measurements are calculated to provide a more accurate (though still not infallible) way to determine if a person is truly over-fat—that is, obese. But the BMI itself is really not an appropriate guide for gauging your child's weight, because it was developed with adults in mind, not children, and the standard adult BMI calculations are not reliable for kids who are less than 5 feet tall.

And even for adults using the BMI, there's no hard and fast number that clearly marks where obesity begins. In fact, there's some disagreement among experts as to where "normal weight" ends. Some say that a BMI anywhere above 25 signifies overweight, whereas former Surgeon General C. Everett Koop (now head of "Shape Up America") sets 27 as the upper limit for normal weight.

There seems to be general agreement, however, that a BMI of 30 usually means obesity, but even that number is a little misleading. Early maturation, genetics, and ethnicity can all cause a higher-than-average BMI. Children who appear to be of normal weight can nonetheless have unhealthy body-fat levels. In fact, a large-scale study conducted by the National Research Council followed 979 boys and girls aged 3 to 18. Preliminary findings of that study showed that 1 out of 6 children who have "normal" BMIs actually have an unhealthy level of body fat.

The thing to keep in mind is that if your child weighs 20 percent or more over the expected weight for a particular height, chances are the child is obese. If your child is very muscular and athletic, of course, that may make a difference.

THE HIGH COSTS OF OBESITY

As I said at the start of this chapter, obesity not only causes problems by increasing your child's risk of disease, it also has an equally devastating effect on their emotional health. The damage, both physical and emotional, takes a huge toll on our kids, and we need to do our best to help them.

Emotional Costs

Remember, obesity means, purely and simply, being overly fat. And it's not fun being fat, especially for a young child. Prejudice against obesity in society in general is evident everywhere you look, from the way overweight people are presented in the media, to the fact that they're even paid less. Did you know that obese white women earn significantly less than their slender counterparts in similar positions? Or that in a survey of 81 employers, nearly half—44 percent—considered obesity a good enough reason to pass over candidates for jobs, claiming that obesity is too much of a medical liability to chance?

That's the "grown-up" version of prejudice against obesity. For kids, there are different, but no less devastating problems. People stare. You have to get your clothes in the "husky" department (and every kid knows what *that* means). And, because kids stigmatize their peers at a very early age, other kids make fun of you. Obese kids are often the victims of teasing or outright bullying by other kids, and they are prime targets for gibes, jokes, and ugly names.

And the situation can become self-perpetuating. Overweight and obese kids are generally not physically active. This may be, in part, by choice, but there's also the fact that fat kids are often left out of sports altogether—nobody wants the "fatty" on *their* team. So they end up with fewer opportunities to get the exercise they need to lose weight, (or to at least prevent any further weight gain) and get into better physical condition. And gym class is often an excruciating exercise in humiliation, not muscles. If the other kids make disparaging comments or the gym teacher is insensitive, the result is a steady erosion of self-esteem, social exclusion, and, often, depression. Not to mention the fact that such children are likely to respond to these bad feelings about themselves by adopting self-destructive behaviors, including dysfunctional eating.

What's worse, childhood and adolescent obesity is a problem that usually doesn't just go away. Not only do all the health risks associated with obesity continue on into adult life, the chances are high that the obesity itself will continue as well. It's an unfortunate fact that the earlier the onset of obesity, the greater the chance of adult obesity, and the long-term health complications are likely to be more severe. How likely is this? Consider these startling facts:

- 25% of obese preschoolers are likely to be obese as adults!

- 75% of obese 12 year olds are likely to be obese as adults!

- 90% of obese adolescents are likely to be obese as adults!

If you're child is obese, you must act *NOW*!

Health Costs

The risks attached to overweight and obesity in children are many, and they can last a lifetime. For example, obese children are subject to the risk factors associated with cardiovascular disease. They're 53 times more likely than their non-obese peers to develop hyperlipidemia—high levels of cholesterol and triglycerides in their blood. They're also more likely to suffer from high blood pressure and insulin resistance. With insulin resistance, the body is unable to control it's blood glucose levels efficiently because the excess fat cells make it harder for the body to respond to insulin— the "key" which allows glucose to enter the cells to be used for energy. Insulin resistance is a major risk factor associated with Type 2 diabetes mellitis—the seventh leading cause of death in the United States.

It's no coincidence that as obesity increases among our children, so do the number of kids suffering from Type 2 diabetes, which used to be prevalent only in adults (and in fact was at one time called "adult" or "mature onset" diabetes). In 1990, less than 4 percent of the diabetes cases in children were of Type 2, now it's 20 percent! The increase is especially pronounced in 10 to 19 year olds.

It's one thing to read statistics like this, but it's even more disturbing when you see it in real life. Believe me! I've been in practice almost 20 years, and until 5 years ago I *never* saw a client under the age of 40 who had Type 2 diabetes. Today I see at least two under-20-year-old patients each week who are dealing with the disease! I've seen all the debilitating complications that Type 2 diabetes can lead to, and when I think of what these kids are at risk for, it honestly frightens me.

What are the medical implications of obesity and Type 2 diabetes? There are plenty. First, children suffering from obesity commonly experience orthopedic problems, especially in the back and in the knees. They are more likely to suffer from asthma and other respiratory problems. They're also likely to have real problems getting fit, because the physical problems just mentioned, and obesity itself, make it difficult to be active. And many children with Type 2 diabetes are malnourished. Even though they may appear to be eating a high-calorie diet, their bodies are not able to properly assimilate the nutrients if their blood sugar is not under control.

Obese children also run an increased risk of developing heart disease as adults. Obese children have higher cholesterol, triglycerides, and blood pressure rates. Combine this with Type 2 diabetes, which by itself increases the risk of heart disease, and you have the recipe for disaster. There's actually a name for this combination of conditions—Syndrome X, which includes hyperlipidemia (high cholesterol), hypertension (high blood pressure), obesity and Type 2 diabetes. The longer a person lives with these conditions, the greater the odds that he or she will suffer with cardiovascular disease and the complications associated with Type 2 diabetes, later in life.

Another medical effect of obesity is the increased likelihood of early maturation. Even *Time* magazine has noted the recent phenomenon that kids today are maturing far earlier than ever. In the October 30, 2000 issue, *Time* ran an article titled "Teens Before Their Time," in which author Michael D. Lemonick reported that a significant number of elementary school girls are developing more mature bodies, with budding breasts and pubic hair. In fact, according to Lemonick, the rise in early-maturation among females is startling: 1 in 7 Caucasian girls start developing breasts and pubic hair by the age of 8; among African-American schoolgirls of that age, the rate is 1 in 2!

This is a physically troubling situation. Early maturation that accompanies obesity is linked with an increased risk for certain types of cancer, including breast cancer. This could be due to the effect of fat on estrogen—excess fat raises estrogen levels, and the longer a woman is exposed to high estrogen levels, the greater her risk of breast cancer. In addition, early maturation and obesity, and particularly the sedentary lifestyle associated with obesity, have been linked to an increased risk of certain cancers later in life.

Social Costs

All these physical problems have a high social and emotional cost for children. To take one obvious example, imagine being an 8 year old girl suddenly undergoing all the physical and hormonal changes associated with puberty. Puberty is often stressful enough for young girls even when it happens at a more expected age. (This is especially true for those among the first of their peers to show noticeable signs of maturing.) Much younger children lack the emotional resources to handle the changes their bodies are going through. It can be devastating!

But even if you ignore for a moment the medical issues—something I do not advise you to do—the fact is that obesity is socially and emotionally damaging in its own right. Obese kids face discrimination from their peers and teachers. They frequently suffer from poor self-esteem and many become socially isolated. Deeply unhappy, they often turn to emotional eating, which only fuels a vicious cycle and adds to their weight.

THEORIES OF OBESITY

The astronomical rise in obesity, among children, has many researchers and health professionals across the country, asking "Why?" As yet doctors have not identified a single, definitive culprit for obesity, but several theories have been developed.

Learned Behavior

Proponents of the learned behavior theory lay a lot of the blame on the child's social environment. They're quick to point out that obese children often have obese parents and they suggest that the child develops dysfunctional eating and poor fitness-related habits by learning from the people around them. In other words, if the parents tend to eat emotionally, or eat a lot of unhealthy foods, the kids are likely to pick up these behaviors, too. And if parents are inactive, their children also tend to be sedentary. The problem is that, true or not, obesity *does* seem to be something that repeats itself across generations—so obese children are likely to grow up to have obese kids of their own!

Fat Cells

The fat-cell theory holds that the number of fat cells in your body determines whether or not you're likely to become obese. In other words, the development of too many fat cells during childhood creates a lifelong weight problem. It's based on two facts of physical development: the body is *always* capable of creating new fat-storage cells, but once those fat cells are created, they never go away—they can only shrink in size.

Here's how it works. As the body increases in weight, fat cells are created to store the excess fuel (calories) your body consumes. Since fat cells prefer to be full rather than empty, they'll fill up whenever they can. Once they're full, if you're still over-eating, new fat cells will form to provide storage for the excess material. If you succeed in losing weight temporarily, the fat cells shrink in size, but their number stays constant. And they're always looking to fill themselves up again, which is why it's so hard to lose weight and so easy to gain it back.

Set Points

Related to the fat-cell theory is the idea that we all have an innate mechanism that programs our bodies to remain at a certain weight. This "programmed weight" is called the "set point." When we cut calories, this innate mechanism increases our appetite and lowers our metabolic rate (and maybe our energy level) in order to force the body back to its preferred weight—the set point. There may be some truth to this set-point idea, but you can't use it as an excuse for obesity. It's highly unlikely that your body would "naturally" prefer a weight that was clearly dangerous for your health. Your natural set point, in other words, is probably a healthy body weight, not a level of obesity.

By the way, it appears that the set point—understood as the weight your body tends to gravitate towards even when you try to lose weight—can be manipulated. Dr. Richard Kesey, a researcher at the University of Wisconsin at Madison, has noted that regular exercise can gradually raise your body's normal metabolic rate, which has the effect of lowering your set point.

Genetics

Experts believe that there are at least 30 to 40 genes that can increase a person's propensity to become obese. That's one reason why the children of obese parents are much more likely to become obese themselves—70 to 80 percent more likely, in fact. Even if only one parent is obese, the chance of a child becoming obese is between 40 to 50 percent. Compare this to the child of two normal-weight parents; this child only runs a 7 percent chance of becoming obese.

But heredity is only one part of the story. After all, children of obese parents get more than just their genes from Mom and Dad. They also get exposure to certain patterns of eating and activity that also predispose them to obesity. And the genetic aspect of obesity can be countered by proper nutrition and an increase in activity levels. In other words, it's *not* an inescapable fate.

A Little of Each

In the fields of nutrition and fitness, many of us believe that the real answer to the question "Why do kids become obese?" can be found in a combination of all 4 theories. Sure, biology and heredity play a role, but they account for approximately 30 percent of the risk of obesity. The other 70 percent of the risk is most likely environmental and therefore controllable. This is important, because it's just too easy to blame obesity on "fat genes" and give up—especially since this means accepting all the health risks that go along with it. For our kids' sake and for future generations, we have to take a firm stand against obesity right now!

WHAT TO DO?

With all its adverse affects on your child's health, and the damage it does to a young child's developing self-esteem, it's clearly important to find a way to help your child overcome this condition—or, better still, to keep it from occurring in the first place. But that means you've got quite a job ahead of you.

The cultural messages that push us all to eat unhealthy foods and to Super Size our fast-food are aimed directly at your kids. So are the subtle and not-so-subtle messages urging that they should eat not because they're hungry but because a nifty toy comes with the meal, or because they're at the movies and everyone has popcorn at the movies—or for emotional reasons. How many TV sit-coms show smart, attractive women race for the gallon of ice cream in the freezer when they break up with their boyfriends? It's a standard joke, treating this as funny but oh-so-normal.

So what *can* you do to help your overweight or obese child? You can't isolate your kids from the unhealthy nutrition messages in the media, and you're probably going to find that your child finds the situation too humiliating to talk comfortably with you about it. On top of which, sometimes we, as parents, aggravate the problem by not recognizing it for what it really is: a health issue that needs to be addressed. Here are some specific steps for dealing with childhood obesity that I've developed over the years in my practice.

1. **Look to yourself, first.** This means taking an honest look at your own attitudes toward food and weight, and identify the ones that may be feeding into your child's obesity. I'm not trying to lay all the blame on you—I know that no parent wishes this on their children. But sometimes we send our children the wrong messages without even realizing it. Remember, parents are the most influential role models in our children's lives!

For example, do *you* turn to food for emotional comfort? You can bet your child sees this and learns to copy your behavior, no matter what you say against it. Do you frequently decide that, after a hectic day, you'd rather grab some quick take-out from a fast-food joint than cook a meal? It's understandable in these hectic times to occasionally take that route, but most fast-food places serve more fat and sugar than anything else, and you're teaching your child that this is a perfectly acceptable substitute for a more conventional meal.

Do you look in the mirror and obsess about your own weight, or poke fun at the weight of your spouse? Your child will notice and begin to internalize your own negative attitudes. What's more, your negative apprehension about your own weight may lead you to misdiagnose your child as overweight or obese when he or she really is not! This is a problem I see often in my own practice— overly weight-conscious parents sometimes seem to be actively *looking* for something to be wrong with their children's bodies! Please don't!!!

2. **Never make an issue of your child's weight.** And never *ever* refer to your child as chubby, husky, or fat—not even jokingly. Kids know the code words. They know that the "husky" department in the clothing store is really the fat-kids section. You may be trying to make light of their weight with a humorous reference to their chubbiness, but they won't hear your intention—they'll only hear the words, which are extremely hurtful to their self-esteem. Ideally, you should never discuss your child's weight in front of him (or her) unless he brings it up himself!!! Of course, if that does happen, you can use it as an opportunity to talk openly and reassuringly on the subject. You can teach about healthful foods, and about the importance of keeping active. And above all, make sure they know that you are there for them, should they seek your support.

3. **Realize that your child's body is not yours.** Everybody's shape is different, because everybody gets a unique pattern from the family gene pool. Some kids are naturally bigger than others of their age. So *NEVER* compare your child to other children—not even to their own brothers or sisters! That's damaging to their sense of self, even when you do it about issues that have nothing to do with weight. Every child wants to be loved for their unique self—not forced to measure up to everyone else.

4. **Never single out an overweight or obese child for special treatment.** That means don't make him or her eat different

meals from the rest of the family, don't hide the snacks but slip them to your other, "normal weight" children. They'll find out and feel even worse about themselves than they already do. Besides, the best treatment for obesity is good nutrition and healthy activity—something that everybody in the family should be aiming for! So when you're modifying a child's intake, make sure that there's lots of social support—make sure they see that eating healthy is desirable for *everyone.*

5. **Try to identify what cues entice your kids to eat when they're not hungry.** Is it boredom? While watching TV? When they're feeling sad? Then work to eliminate those cues where possible and substitute other things for food when necessary. For example, if they constantly ask for snacks out of boredom, suggest a fun activity instead—you could even play a game with them. That way you get an extra benefit—an unexpected chance to spend a little quality time communicating and building bonds with your child! When you can't eliminate the cue, as when a child doesn't feel well or is sad, take a moment to comfort that child emotionally—maybe sing a song together or, if they're older, encourage them to write about what's troubling them. This way they'll learn new ways to cope with their emotions, without developing an unhealthy relationship with food.

6. **Make a point of keeping very few, if any, high-fat snack foods around.** Such foods should not be a part of *anyone's* daily intake, anyway. A once-in-awhile treat, maybe, but there are plenty of tasty snacks— pretzels, nuts, fresh fruit, and so on—that you can keep on hand instead. And while we're on the subject of snacks, it's good to note that the healthy choices mentioned above are high in fiber, so they'll easily satisfy your child's hungry feeling. Not a bad deal when you realize that they're also chock-full of essential nutrients as well!

7. **Limit "treats" to one a day.** On the other hand, you don't want to make "treats" like candy or chips a forbidden pleasure, because we all know the forbidden is more attractive

simply because it's forbidden! Occasional treats are fine, just don't go overboard. One treat a day should be the norm. Remember, it's all a matter of portion control. And when you give out these occasional treats, remember: *DON'T USE THEM—OR ANY OTHER FOOD—AS REWARDS!* Find non-food rewards, like a trip to the park or the zoo, a movie, or a new toy. Using food as a reward sets a bad example and teaches kids to indulge in emotional eating!

8. **Find out if it's hunger or thirst.** Make a point of checking to see if it's really food your child needs. Lots of kids don't know how to tell the difference between hunger and thirst—they feel an urge for *something* and immediately think of a snack, when they might actually just be thirsty! Offer a drink instead. Plain water is best, but you can add an ounce or two of juice to give it flavor, if that will make it more appealing. But *don't* think that all drinks are created equal. Sodas and juice drinks are definitely *not* your best choice.

9. **Step up the activity.** A big contributor to childhood obesity is childhood *inactivity!* Remember back when you were a kid and your Mom (or Dad) would say "What are you doing hanging around inside, when it's beautiful outside?" Well, it's time to start sounding like your parents! If your children tend to hang around the house, parked in front of the TV or the video games, start setting some limits. If your neighborhood isn't one in which you feel safe letting the kids run around, check your community for alternatives. The important thing is that your child start getting regular physical activity.

10. *NEVER EVER PUT YOUR CHILD ON A DIET!* As a health professional in practice for almost 20 years, I've seen enough evidence to know that diets don't work, not even for adults. So why would anyone expect them to be okay for growing children!?! Not only are diets generally ineffective with kids, they can actually create health problems because they interfere with their nutrient needs and growth. It's much better to help them grow *into* their

weight by teaching healthier lifestyle behaviors, proper nutrition, and a good daily dose of physical activity. We'll take up the subject of dieting in greater detail in the next chapter. Right now, however, just remember: *NEVER* put your child on a diet!

MY STORY

You may have noticed that I have very strong feelings on this subject. Part of this is because my professional work and training have shown me how devastating childhood obesity can be. But I have a much stronger, personal reason for my attitudes.

I was always a heavy child, escalating to 168 pounds at the young age of 14, with only 65 inches of height to my credit! The teasing I took throughout grade school was constant—and occasionally even my family and friends joined in. The teasing hurt, even when there wasn't any malice behind it. I remember how bad it felt to be singled out that way, to have people stare or make pointed comments about my size. To numb the pain that the teasing caused me, I would often secretly turn to food for comfort, which of course just made matters worse.

I dreaded changing into shorts and a T-shirt to participate in gym class. I wanted to fit in with the other kids, but those skimpy gym suits the teacher forced us to wear gave me no way to hide my excess weight. When I was in 8th grade, I even had to have a seamstress tailor-make a cheerleading uniform for me, because I couldn't fit into the regular ones that the school handed out! The embarrassment was *excruciating*. And when I got to puberty and started wanting boys to like me, I'd feel humiliated when they saw me in those gym shorts!

At home, it seemed like there was no place to turn for support and reassurance. My Mom had spent a lifetime struggling with her own weight, so she couldn't help me. After all, if she never learned to love her own body, how was she to teach me to accept my own? And family members made well-meaning (usually) remarks about my weight, thinking that this would inspire me to slim down—not realizing that all they were doing was confirming my belief that there was something really unacceptable and just plain wrong about me.

This basically erased any sense of self-esteem I had. No matter what I did, no matter how I succeeded in other areas of my life, my weight—and my inability to control it—was all that mattered! This is a terrible way for a child to feel, and it can lead to some really dangerous choices, as you'll learn in the next chapter.

PUTTING THE TIPS INTO PRACTICE

Coping with childhood overweight and obesity is really coping with two things at once, as you probably sensed from the tips I gave earlier. The first is preventative—you want to ensure that a healthy-weight child stays that way. Second is to address any problems that may already have begun. That can seem pretty daunting, but in fact a big part of the solution addresses both situations at once. That's because the best thing you can do in either case is to be aware and start working against obesity as early as possible.

But if obesity is already a problem, don't expect to see immediate changes once you've begun working to overcome it. You need to be patient, because it's a gradual process, and if you're impatient your child will just have one more thing to feel bad about. So the goal is to take it slowly and steadily, and to be as supportive as you possibly can throughout the process. Because that's what's needed right now—a process in which you teach your child the basic principles of designing a healthy lifestyle, not a quick-fix.

For example, if you're working through the tips I've given you, you've begun to pay attention to your own attitudes about weight. You'll have noticed whether or not you unconsciously criticize your body in the mirror or make a big deal about gaining a couple of extra pounds. You may have also caught yourself unknowingly making remarks to your child that can hurt their self-esteem, however good your initial intentions. As you learn to take your own focus off scales and pounds, you'll begin to see your child gradually become less anxious about his or her own weight. And as anxiety levels decrease, your child will become more receptive to other steps that will lead to a healthier weight.

Similarly, as you learn to pay greater attention to how food is treated in your household, you can begin to extinguish some practices that encourage over-eating or the establishment of unhealthy food relationships. You'll begin to learn not to push your children to eat more than he or she really wants, just because you expect them to "clean their plates." You'll learn not to use terms like "bad foods" versus "good foods." And you'll catch yourself before you fall into the trap of using food as a reward.

You'll also be able to help your child address inappropriate food habits, once your child is less stressed-out about his or her weight. This may take some time and effort, because we all know that habits are powerful things—and that they're really hard to break, even when you know a habit is bad for you. If you're starting on a healthy lifestyle plan early in your child's life, you'll have a much easier time than those who start in later years, when the temptation to indulge in poor eating practices gets stronger. But even if your child is already indulging in unhealthy eating habits, all is not lost.

One way to break undesirable habits is to enlist your child in helping to spot them. Of course, this can't be truly effective until you have reached a point when your child is receptive to talking about his or her weight, but if you're supportive and make yourself available, that day will come. You can help it along by involving your child in food preparation for family meals—the time you spend together, and the opportunities this gives you to teach about good nutrition without "getting personal," can begin to open doors for communication. Once those doors are open, you can begin to talk about how *everybody* has unexamined habits about food, and suggest ways to spot them.

A good way to start is by getting your child involved in keeping a "food and mood log." He or she should record the foods eaten each day—*including* drinks and snacks—and how it felt to consume them. You can do this even with little kids, using pictures instead of words—the important thing is to match the tool with the child's level of development. The following chart shows how a log like this would look for a child of around the age of 10.

If you're also teaching about balanced meals, you can use these logs to help your child figure out where better choices could be made—both food choices or picking an activity other than eating. Are they getting enough fruits and veggies each day? Are they varying their carbohydrates or only eating breads and crackers? This kind of self-monitoring is good for kids, because it lets them feel as if they have some control over their lives. It also lets them become more aware of their own behaviors and allows them to see real achievements over time. Remember, the goal isn't really weight loss—it's developing healthy habits to prevent further

Time of Day	Food and Drink	Amount	Food Category	Hunger Level	Activity While Eating	Mood
9am	scrambled egg English muffin butter skim milk	1 1 whole 1 tsp 1 cup	1 meat 2 grains 1 fat (extra) 1 dairy	3	sitting	tired
12pm	sandwich: sliced wheat bread turkey breast mayo lettuce and tomatoes apple skim chocolate milk	2 slices 2 slices 1 tsp a few slices 1 1 cup	2 grains 1 meat (2 oz) 1 fat 2 veggies 1 fruit 1 dairy	4	at school	okay
3pm	pretzels bottle of water	about 20 20 oz	1.5 grains extra	3	watching tv	bored
6pm	chicken leg cooked carrots mashed potatoes applesauce water	1 2 scoops (1 cup) a big pile (1 cup) 1 scoop (1 cup) big glass	1 meat (3 oz) 2 veggies 2 grains 1 fruit extra	4	eating with family	tired
8pm	ice cream cone	1 scoop 1 cone	1 dairy 1/2 grain	2	watching tv	tired

weight gain. The good news is that if your child is obese, these same healthy habits will actually work to gradually bring him or her down to a healthy weight!

When trying to help children make lasting changes, it's best to allow them to make some decisions for themselves. As parents, we need to set the stage for better choices—in particular, by making sure that more healthy foods are readily available, and by setting a good example by our own behaviors. Over time, we *can* teach our children to listen to their bodies and help them to end the dysfunctional behaviors that lead to obesity. *AND* we can do this without starting them on the self-defeating cycle of a lifetime of "yo-yo" dieting!

STRATEGIES FOR SUCCESS

Setting the stage for your child's success in beating childhood obesity *IS* within your grasp. Here are some tactics that you'll find helpful:

1. **Enlist total family involvement and a positive support system.** At least one parent must be interested and involved in order for there to be success, but it's best to have the whole family involved. Eat the same foods that you prepare for your overweight or obese child, so there's no stigma attached, and exercise together so that it doesn't appear to be a punishment. The added benefit is that the whole family will end up healthier and will develop healthy lifestyle habits all at the same time!

2. **Make mealtime a pleasant experience.** The obvious thing is to avoid mealtime arguments and stressful conversations. And forbid TV watching while eating—in fact, make it a rule that the TV is turned off! Even having it as background noise is disruptive: there's nothing more stressful than a loud cartoon or the news blaring, while you're trying to have a nice, relaxing family meal. And there are other helpful things you can do. For example, you can establish a minimum time for meals—at least 30 minutes is good, no matter what the meal (including breakfast), because it allows time to eat slowly and really appreciate the food. Eating slowly also gives your child a chance to realize

when he or she has had enough, whereas rushing a meal often results in overeating—the body doesn't have time to figure out that it's full!

3. **No more "family style" service.** Putting out serving platters full of food encourages over-eating. It's much better to serve individual portions on plates, instead. When everybody serves themselves, you often get the "eyes are bigger than the stomach" syndrome: taking a huge portion, then feeling obligated to eat the whole thing just because it's on your plate. Serving portions, on the other hand, allows you to avoid this problem. If your child truly is still hungry after the first portion, he or she can go back for seconds perhaps, but it will now be a conscious choice. In fact, I recommend setting a "15-minute rule" for seconds: wait 15 minutes after finishing one serving before going back for more. That gives the belly enough time to let the brain know if it's had enough. And while we're on the subject of portion control, do the same thing with snacks. Buy single-serving snacks, or if you buy in bulk, take the time to re-package the food into single portions. It's just too easy to grab that "jumbo" bag of chips and eat the whole thing absent-mindedly, but if the snacks are only available in individual portions, the temptation to overindulge is much less.

4. **Involve your kids in meal preparation.** Overweight kids are often discouraged from the kitchen, but this is a strategy that can backfire. First of all, it increases the allure of food as something restricted or forbidden. Second, it makes it harder to teach your children about healthy foods, meal planning, portion control, and so on. On the other hand, if a child is involved in preparing the meal—say, cutting and preparing the veggies and arranging them attractively on the plates—he or she will feel the pride of accomplishment and might be just that much more likely to eat the healthful foods.

5. **Make healthy living fun.** Put a little effort into making foods look attractive and interesting on the plate—after all, you'd do as much if you were entertaining company,

wouldn't you? A visually stimulating meal is just as inviting as one that smells good. Similarly, add an element of fun to exercise—family bike rides, a rousing game of Frisbee in the backyard, a hiking trip, or even just dancing around the living room. Fun activities are much more likely to tempt your sedentary child into action.

6. **Get your child *involved*.** Your child must have a personal interest in having a healthier lifestyle. Meal planning and preparation, selecting family activities, even going along to the grocery store, are all areas where your child can play a role. This is especially important if other family members tend to favor competitive sports over non-competitive activities, because an overweight or obese child will often avoid such situations and sit the game out on the sidelines. If your overweight child has some say in the matter, however, he or she can choose something that they're good at. Children need to feel competent, and giving them the opportunity to make some decisions is a great way to boost this feeling.

7. **Know your respective roles.** You and your child may be working together toward the goal of developing a healthy lifestyle, but each of you has a different role to play. Your role is to have healthful foods on hand, to prepare proper portions at meals, and to establish some controls and limits. In addition, you just have to be a good parent: providing a supportive, loving environment in which your child can develop a sense of himself or herself as valuable and well loved. Your child's role is to discover what his or her body is really saying, and to learn to respond to it appropriately.

Remember, the more we expose our children to healthy habits, the more likely they'll internalize and adopt these good behaviors as their own. And after all, the only true and lasting remedy for childhood obesity is the rejection of unhealthy lifestyle habits and the adoption of healthy ones in their place. Sure it would be wonderful if society at large—the schools, the community, the media —would cooperate in this goal, but that's not likely to happen anytime soon. So it's up to *you*. Only you can put your child on the right path, and only you can provide the inspiration and example your child really needs.

IS THERE A DIETER IN THE HOUSE?

9

$\mathcal{O}$verweight and obesity in children and teens often leads to dieting. Sometimes it's the parents who prompt the diet, sometimes children will try to do it on their own. And sometimes, sadly enough, medical doctors who should know better, actually recommend that the child be put on a diet. But this is rarely an appropriate action to take. Today's health and nutrition professionals largely agree that dieting doesn't work. Dieting encourages dysfunctional eating habits and forces it's victims to obsess about restricted foods and the numbers on the scale, rather than putting the focus where it should be—on achieving good health.

WHY DIETING DOESN'T WORK

The word "diet" can be confusing. We talk about "a balanced diet" when what we really mean is a meal plan, and then we talk about "going on a diet" when we mean restricting our food intake in order to lose weight. When I say "dieting doesn't work," I'm talking about the latter: *restrictive dieting*.

The human body is designed to survive. It needs the food we eat in order to perform all sorts of functions, from distributing nutrients through the blood, permitting our nervous systems and senses to operate, repairing and replacing layers of skin which naturally slough off daily—and everything from breathing to muscle building. If we don't consume adequate amounts of calories and nutrients, the body will make do with what it has, becoming more efficient in using that energy.

What does this mean in weight maintenance terms? It means slowing the metabolism and burning less calories than normal. But when the food restriction (the diet) ends, and you return to your previous eating behavior (the one that caused you to gain the excess weight in the first place), you gain the weight right back! Here's how it works:

You decrease your intake to lose weight. Then, after a few weeks, the weight doesn't seem to drop anymore, because your body is looking out for its survival, so it cuts back on it's use of fuel (calories). This is the "plateau" that dieters talk about. Your body hits this plateau so that it can evaluate whether or not its fluids, electrolytes, and other vital nutrients are still in balance, but most dieters respond to this temporary peak by cutting their intake even *more*! That's when the real trouble begins!

After awhile, most dieters slip "off the wagon" and splurge, and this is usually followed by a period when they slip back into their old eating habits. Then, all of a sudden, the weight comes back! And every time this diet/deprivation-splurge cycle occurs, you lose lean body weight that *doesn't* come back! For example, lets imagine a 20-year-old woman who weighs 190 pounds. She goes on a few diets during her adulthood, but never really makes a permanent change in her weight (this is typical). By the time she is a 45-year-old woman, she still weighs 190 pounds, but the percentage of body fat in that weight is *much* higher than it was when she was 20!

What does this mean to a dieter? First of all, it means that if your body can't find enough fuel (glucose) floating freely in the blood stream, it will look for another alternative. It's first choice as an energy substitute is glycogen—your body's stored form of carbohydrates, which is kept in muscle tissue and the liver. This glycogen will be broken down into glucose and dispersed into the blood as needed, where it will be taken up by cells for their energy needs. If the deprivation continues, the body will eventually turn to the protein in your muscle tissue. Muscle tissue includes everything from the biceps and triceps in the upper arms to a person's heart, liver, and kidneys (yes, your organs are also made of muscle tissue). At the same time, your body continues to reduce it's energy needs, which results in a further decrease in your ability to burn calories (your metabolism). The result? You continue to burn fewer calories everyday—which makes it much easier to put weight back on again.

At the same time, dieting is essentially an exercise in self-deprivation and food obsession. In order to follow a diet, you need to be thinking about food all the time—constantly aware of which foods are "permitted" and which are "forbidden." But it's human nature for a forbidden object to become an obsession. We start craving it, and it becomes almost impossible to stop thinking about it. This is especially true if the forbidden item is something we find pleasurable—like food. It's no different than my 7-year-old son and his playthings. If I set him up in a room with 100 of his favorite toys and point to one toy and say "you can play with anything but that one," guess which one he wants?

THE DANGERS OF DIETING FOR THE YOUNG

Everything negative that we've discovered about dieting in general is even more detrimental for growing children, whose bodies are still developing. Restricting a child's calorie intake means the child will be getting fewer nutrients than their bodies need for proper development. To make matters worse, enforcing a restrictive diet on a child can have serious emotional consequences as well, and usually leads to a loss of self-confidence, self-esteem, and a poor sense of self.

These emotional factors can't be emphasized strongly enough. Obsession with food, feelings of low self-esteem, and distorted body images, all contribute to setting our children up for yo-yo dieting and a negative sense of self that can plague them throughout their lives. And the impact of this is especially pronounced on kids who are too young to truly understand *why* they're being singled out and restricted.

Children start out with a pretty good sense of self—even when they have to deal with serious problems like disfigurement or disability. They don't automatically blame *themselves* for their condition, until somebody starts to suggest that it's somehow their fault! And that's what dieting tells a child—that their body is unacceptable, and so are *they!* Obviously, this can do tremendous damage to self esteem, and it will trickle down through every part of that child's life! They can easily start believing that they're not good enough, not smart enough, not worthy enough—so why try to do *anything* at all!

As I've said before, putting kids on diets is rarely a good idea—it should happen only rarely, when a diagnosed illness requires specific food restrictions. Such illnesses might include gluten enteropathy or Celiac's disease, in which they can't process the gluten in wheat and other grains. But the restriction here has nothing to do with weight loss—it's an avoidance of food that the body simply can't process correctly. There are also some childhood diseases, like phenylketonuria (PKU), which was mentioned in regards to aspartame, in which kids can't process phenylalanine, a specific amino acid, so they have to avoid all foods that contain it.

THE DO-IT-YOURSELF DILEMMA

By now it should be clear that parents and doctors should not put kids on diets, if the only health problem is the excess weight. But what about when kids decide to "do it themselves" and begin dieting on their own. Kids, especially teenagers, are susceptible to fads and fashions, and they're bombarded with ads for Slim Fast and Weight Watchers on TV, not to mention the print ads in magazines aimed directly at kids and teens. But kids are usually unprepared to truly investigate a diet's claims—or its dangers. Nor do they care if it's dangerous—their ultimate goal is to fit in with their peers at whatever costs, so they're unlikely to pay much attention to the health warnings that show up in small print at the bottom of the TV screen or the print ads. And kids are impatient for results, so they're much more likely to fall for programs that offer "quick weight loss" or bill themselves as "miracle" diets.

Dangerous Fads

There seems to be no end to the variety of "miracle" diets that are being pushed on the public. They all have one thing in common: they promise weight loss with little effort and in a very short amount of time. In fact, though, they all tend to fall into just a few general categories. The following fad diets are likely to cause the greatest damage.

High-protein/low-carbohydrate diets. The most famous of these is the Atkins diet—also known medically as the ketogenic diet. I call it the "all you can eat of steak, eggs, and cheese but God forbid you get a whiff of carbohydrates" diet. The high-protein (which means high fat and high cholesterol) content of this diet can't be healthy when you think about how excess fat and cholesterol are related to an increased risk of heart disease. And with the restriction on carbohydrates, how can you get the nutrients that come from whole grains, fruits and veggies!?

The low carbohydrate content of these diets means low glucose—so these diets quickly result in glucose deprivation. But glucose is what the body prefers as fuel, so it has to find an alternative source. What it uses is protein and fat. However, when a protein is turned into a glucose molecule, it leaves nitrogen molecules behind. The nitrogen molecules join to form ammonia and urea, which your body has to filter out through the kidneys. And your body builds up ketones as it burns up fat, so it needs to draw fluid from the cells to flush the ketones out of your kidneys, too. (That's why the early weight loss is so high on these diets—you're losing lots of body water, NOT body fat!) This can lead to dehydration and electrolyte imbalance if you stay on the diet for more than a few weeks at a time. Meanwhile, your kidneys are working overtime. Think of the kidney as a spaghetti strainer—it can strain small particles out, but larger, harsher particles like ammonia, urea, and ketones get caught. This can eventually cause irreversible kidney damage.

Also, the high fat and cholesterol content often leads to increases in the dieter's bad cholesterol (LDL) and triglycerides. I have personally had more than a handful of patients referred to me for high cholesterol after following a ketogenic diet. And this diet also leads to an increased calcium loss from bones. This is because protein is high in phosphorus, which competes with calcium for absorption into the body, and calcium often loses. (Diet sodas cause a similar problem, by the way, because of their high phosphorus content!)

Very low fat diets. Diets that go overboard in cutting out fats mean that your child or teen is getting too few fat soluble vitamins —A, D, E, and K—and essential fatty acids. But fats are vital; they're a part of all cell membranes, including the neurons, a significant part of the nervous system and the brain cells. Deprive the brain of these fatty acids and the brain cells simply can't function properly. Deprive them long enough, and some of those neurons will die. And, of course, it's easy to end up taking in too few calories with this type of diet, leading to the loss of body protein and a lowered metabolism.

All-fruit or vegetable diets or juicing fasts. These include the old "grapefruit diet" and the so-called Beverly Hills diet. Beyond the obvious fact that such diets mean depriving the body of necessary protein and fat, these "one food group" diets are devoid of numerous other nutrients. Unfortunately, the majority of weight lost with this type of fad diet is water, which typically leaves the body in the form of diarrhea. Now that's not exactly what I would call a comfortable—or healthy—way to lose weight. The end result is basically nothing more than dehydration. Drink some fluids to replenish your body and that "lost weight" comes right back!

In addition, single-food diets—and even restrictive diets like the Atkins high-protein approach—are *boring*? There's only so much of a single food or food group that you can eat with enjoyment. These diets often subtly count on this fact—they figure that if there's no pleasure in eating, you'll tend to eat less. The problem is that you're just as likely to start obsessing about the foods you're not allowed to eat, which guarantees that you'll fall off your diet, regain the weight, and feel like a failure.

Very low-calorie diets. Extremely low calorie diets (under 1,000 calories per day), even if they're more or less balanced in regards to their proportions of protein, carbohydrates, and fat, are not ample enough in energy for the body to perform top notch. This extremely restrictive type of diet doesn't allow for much of *any* foods. Without enough calories to burn, the body begins to go into the starvation mode. That means your metabolism slows down and you begin to burn muscle protein for fuel, leaving you too weak and too tired to do much of anything.

These diets are usually based on a liquid fast—little solid food, mostly a diet drink of some sort. The drink is supposed to have enough nutrients to keep you going, but only barely. One of their operating principles is that they cause a "break" in your normal eating behavior—supposedly so you can stop indulging in dysfunctional or compulsive eating. Instead, you don't have to think about food at all—you just open a can or a package and you're set. The problem is that they don't teach you what to do when you've finished with the program—they don't offer you new, healthier eating habits to replace your old, dysfunctional ones. So when you've lost the weight and are ready to go back to regular meals, you're also likely to go back to the same old eating behaviors and gain the weight right back—and then some!

In fact, very low calorie diets are extremely dangerous to try on your own. They should always be medically monitored, with blood tests done every two weeks to monitor your electrolytes. Don't let the "liquid" in the title fool you, these diets can lead to serious dehydration and electrolyte imbalance. They can lead to cardiac arrythmia and, ultimately, cardiac arrest. But even if you avoid these dire results, less severe side effects include nausea, bad breath, a foul-scented perspiration (thanks to the ketones produced, it smells like ammonia and apples), low blood sugar, lethargy, and dry skin! Clearly, no child should *EVER* be put on this kind of diet—*EVER!*

In my work, I've seen people try to make up their own version of a liquid fast. Teens are apt to try something like this because they just don't realize the potential danger they're facing. They just figure "If 2 cans of diet drink plus a meal are good, 3 cans and skipping the meal will be better, right?" Next thing you know, you've got a pretty sick child on your hands!

Pre-packaged, frozen-meal programs. Think Weight Watchers and Smart Ones. The biggest problem here is that these frozen entrees are awfully expensive and usually not very tasty. On top of that, they don't really teach people how to take control of their portions or to balance their nutrients. And if you never learn how to do that, you're stuck eating pre-portioned frozen dinners forever! It's far better to learn to serve proper portions and make your own tasty meals.

Nutrient Deprivation

One thing that all these diets have in common is that they restrict your intake—usually by limiting you to one or a few food types. We already know that adults on diets run serious health risks, especially if they go on a diet without a doctor's supervision, so it stands to reason that kids can be damaged too. The problem is, we don't know just *how bad* the risks are to kids, because no experimental studies are ever designed to use children as "guinea pigs." It violates every code of scientific ethics. Still, certain conclusions can be drawn, just based on what we know about how the body works.

Basically, gradual weight loss is okay for kids or for adults, so long as it is combined with exercise to maintain a lean body. However, strict dieting necessarily leads to inadequate nutrient intake. With kids, the main nutrient concerns are protein, calcium, iron, and zinc—all of which are likely to be lacking because dairy and beef, the best sources for these nutrients, are thought to be "fattening." The anemia that results from inadequate iron leads to poor oxygen supply to the muscles and organs, including the brain, and to inadequate red blood cell formation.

Next, too little calorie intake means a slower metabolism, but it also leads to a less effective immune system, leaving dieting kids far more susceptible to infection and far less able to fight it off! And as the body starts consuming lean body mass, the heart muscle itself can be a victim. This leads to decreased blood volume, low blood pressure, and a depressed heart rate.

There are also hormonal changes associated with consuming too few calories. The thyroid and parathyroid glands don't function as accurately as they should. This can cause cold intolerance, especially in the extremities because they're furthest away from the heart. This cold intolerance is also due to the loss of insulation that body fat provides, and to the lowered metabolism that comes with "starvation mode." And since the thyroid plays a role in brain development as well, you really don't want children to be messing with a diet that compromises the functioning of their minds!

Very low calorie diets also disturb the function of the pituitary gland, which regulates the fluid balance in your body. It also affects the pancreas, which secrets insulin and glucagon, both of which are needed to regulate blood sugar levels (energy). Your child could end up with an electrolyte imbalance, too, and this can be fatal. After all, electrolytes help regulate muscle contraction—including the heart! An imbalance could lead to cardiac arrest! That's why doctors are supposed to closely monitor people on liquid diets.

Diet-induced dehydration can cause constipation, because there's less fluid to combine with the feces for easy elimination. It can also cause muscle cramping, dizziness, lightheadedness, and "foggy" thinking. None of which are conditions you'd really want for yourself, let alone your child. And inadequate calorie intake can lead to gastrointestinal problems too. The stomach keeps pumping out hydrochloric acid to break down food, but if there's no food in the belly, it will eat at the stomach lining instead, leading to ulcers. If it backs up into the mouth (in the saliva), it will decay the teeth, too!

With the hormonal changes caused by dieting, young women also face the problem of amenorrhea. This means that they stop having their periods. This may be caused in part because the body knows it's too starved to successfully support a fetus, so it shuts the system down. After all, fat storage around the (mother's) abdomen is important for fetal growth. Female dieters also have to cope with a decrease in estrogen production. This in turn leads to increased calcium loss, which sets the stage for osteoporosis.

On top of all these effects of nutrient deprivation are the more noticeable but less drastic symptoms. Among these are irritability, mood swings, fatigue, and lethargy. Not to mention dark circles under the eyes, dry skin, brittle nails, dull hair—and possibly even hair *loss!*

WHEN PARENTS SUPERVISE DIETS

As you can see, kids who embark on unsupervised diets run the risk of numerous health problems down the road. As adults, they will be more likely to suffer from maladies, such as osteoporosis. They will also be more likely to suffer the effects of a slowed metabolism—which may eventually affect thyroid function. Since the thyroid is involved in creating some of the hormones needed for reproduction, this can have an adverse effect on fertility.

But the problems can still be there, even when a child diets under supervision. If the parents are not fully educated about nutrition, they can make mistakes that put the child at risk of the same health problems we've just finished discussing. On top of which, diets that are imposed on kids by their parents usually backfire. After all, forbidden foods just become much more attractive —you pretty much guarantee that the child is going to want them more than ever.

Imposing a diet on your child also raises serious issues about control. Take complete control over your child's food intake, and you essentially undermine your child's ability to develop self-control and a healthy attitude to his or her food and appetite. This can backfire in two different ways. For some kids, your control over their intake will mean that they'll never learn to pay attention to their own hunger and satiety signals. For other, more rebellious types, you're setting up a constant battle-ground at mealtimes. Either way, you're bound to create a dysfunctional eater.

As if things weren't bad enough, when a parent puts a child on a restrictive diet and is closely involved in administering the intake, the child can't help but feeling as if he's constantly under the gleaming eye of "the food police," always being judged. This is devastating for a child's fragile self-esteem! If you've been on any kind of diet yourself, just think about how it felt when someone noticed your food intake and said, "should you be eating that?" or "don't you think you had enough?" You know how embarrassed and resentful it made you feel—and your child will feel exactly the same way.

Finally, there's the problem of inevitable failure and how that can affect your child's self-esteem. Even grown-ups fall off their diets—a lot—so yes, your child will likely "slip up" and sneak a forbidden treat once in awhile, too. Let's face it, deprivation isn't easy, and no one wants to be told they can't have or do something, so why should we expect children to be any different?

But along with the guilt of sneaking, the child will also likely face powerful feelings of having failed in two ways: failing at the diet, and failing to live up to parental expectations. That's a heavy burden to bear for anyone, especially a child. And the sneaking itself is a bad habit to get into. Sneak-eating now sets the stage for "closet" eating later on—even in adulthood. Believe me, I know—having been under the eyes of many "food cops" myself, I still sometimes feel guilty for eating something out in public when I'm sitting by myself.

And as if all these negatives weren't enough, dieting for children is likely to have some very long-lasting, damaging effects. Dieting establishes an unnatural, deprivation-oriented relationship with food, while at the same time teaching the child to obsess about the numbers on the bathroom scales. What better way to set a child up for eating disorders later on?!

Remember, kids with weight problems didn't get there on their own. Many have been overfed by caretakers all along, and this chronic over-feeding has just finally caught up with them. My own son was overfed for a time, by a caretaker, when he switched from breast to bottled milk. The caretaker routinely added cereal to the bottle because he heard that it would make a child sleep better. Well, sure it would—the poor infant was put into a food coma! The problem is that this kind of early overfeeding causes the child to develop excess fat cells—and you'll remember from the last chapter that those cells never go away!

Since children come by their weight problems through the foods and feeding behaviors they learn from the people around them, it's just plain unfair that they should come to feel that their weight is somehow their own fault! That's why I stress that support, sound nutrition, and healthy—but unforced—activity are the best things you can give your child. They're certainly *lots* better than putting him on a strict diet!

MY LIFE AS A YOUTHFUL DIETER

After years of dealing with my childhood obesity, the adults around me decided to take action. I'll never forget the first diet book I ever got. I was only 12 years old, and it was given to me by my doctor—a 50-year-old, 300 pound pediatrician! He should have *known* better! I'll never forget that day! I can still see that bright yellow booklet with the big, black letters. From that moment on, my life would be very different.

For the next few years, I tried a lot of different weight-loss plans. My family tried to be supportive, and my Mom (who always struggled with her own weight) really understood the pain and frustration I was experiencing. Together we fell into a pattern of dieting together for a few weeks, then "blowing it" with a splurge and giving up. Soon enough, however, we'd start the cycle all over again with a new diet plan—the yo-yo pattern familiar to all chronic dieters. But we never got any closer to our weight-loss goals, and if anything, this pattern just increased our feelings of failure and deprivation.

But diets were just part of the whole problem. There was also the constant sense that I was being watched by the "food police"— everybody seemed to be focused on every little bite I ate. And of course, we got into the whole "good food," "bad food" mentality. Not to mention the "good day," "bad day" trip: if I lost a pound it was a *wondrous* day. If I gained weight or even just stayed the same, I was miserable and anxious. My whole world revolved around what the bathroom scales told me each morning, and there were very few wondrous days in my dieting years.

It wasn't long before the frustration and the constant sense of failure basically killed off any sense of self-worth I had left, and along the way I picked up a lot of really bad attitudes about food and eating. Like a lot of kids who are put on diets at an early age, I was primed and ready to move on to the "big leagues," full-blown eating disorders, as you'll learn in the next chapter.

SPOTTING THE SECRET DIETER

Young children are not immune from "secret" dieting—especially if the parents are always talking about dieting themselves. I see it at my son's parties: little girls who refuse cake or ice cream because it's "fattening." If that's the case in your house, your first priority is to re-evaluate your own attitudes about dieting and weight—kids don't come up with ideas like this on their own. But in general, youngsters are not likely to put themselves on a diet before they hit puberty, for this is the time in their life when the pressures to "fit in" or "look cool" take precedence over everything else.

The trouble is, when children reach puberty they've already begun to have a lot more general autonomy in their lives, so its easier for them to go on a diet without your knowledge than it would be for their younger siblings. Here are some things to watch for that signal your child may be dieting, or may be thinking of doing so in the near future:

- **Changes eating behaviors.** If your child doesn't seem to be eating as much as usual, or has become pickier about foods, you may be seeing the signs of a self-imposed diet. If she seems to be calculating what she eats, or starts limiting her food choices to salads and veggies, chances are high she's dieting.

- **Starts referring to different foods as "good" versus "bad,"** "healthy" versus "unhealthy," or "fattening" versus "safe." (This is self-explanatory.)

- **Denigrates own appearance.** If your child tends to refer to him- or herself as fat, unattractive, or just plain unpopular because of appearances, you're hearing the expression of a bad case of negative body image. Such children are prone to look for "magic" solutions, like miracle diets. And it's just *so* sad to see a beautiful little child look at herself in the mirror and say she's fat or ugly, pointing to a non-existent belly!

- **Denigrates the appearance of others.** This indicates an inappropriate obsession with body shape and size, even if that interest is directed outward, at other people who don't seem to live up to ideal expectations. A child who has such a highly critical attitude toward others can easily turn that criticism on herself.

- **Seems more obsessed with food and mealtimes.** All of a sudden they're interested in what you're making for dinner, and it's only breakfast time! When a child appears to be calculating the day's intake, he's no longer eating for hunger—he's making sure he gets his share. That's a clear sign that food has taken on an inappropriate role and importance to your child.

- **Over-reacts to treats, or refuses treats that she used to enjoy.** Even if a child seems to be eating regular meals, refusing treats may signal the beginnings of a disordered relationship with food, or a growing fixation with weight. Refusing a snack once in awhile shouldn't raise an alarm, but if your child has always liked treats and suddenly starts refusing them regularly, then you may need to take a closer look. Of course, if you've rarely had snacks available, and your children have become accustomed to choosing healthier snacks by preference, they may voluntarily turn down the offer of candy in favor of something like a piece of fruit.

- **Frequently asks to be excused from regular family meals.** A child who's trying to stick to a diet—particularly a very restrictive one—will find it hard to maintain the diet in the face of the more balanced meals the rest of the family eats. Staying away from the table at mealtimes makes it easier to avoid "temptation" and to hide the fact that he is following a very different food regimen. (But this behavior can also be the sign of an even more dangerous eating disorder—as you'll learn in the next chapter.)

- **Breath smells like apple-scented ammonia.** Here's a subtle clue that your child is trying to follow a high protein/low carbohydrate type diet. This very popular fad diet is very dangerous for kids, as we just discussed. It's the kind of diet that causes the body to manufacture ketones to replace the glucose it is no longer getting, as you learned in the section above. It's the ketones that cause the smell of apple-like ammonia on the breath.

BREAKING FREE OF THE DIET CYCLE

We all know people who've tried every diet known to man and still end up regaining the weight, so it shouldn't come as a surprise to learn that diets just *don't work*. Well, if that's the case, why keep trying them. Instead, why not try a whole new approach? After all, what have you got to lose?

And what would this new approach be, you may ask? Bottom line: help your child learn the principles of healthy eating, exercise, and values, as discussed throughout this book. Even an obese child is more likely to benefit from a well-balanced, healthy lifestyle than from a restrictive, weight-obsessed approach to losing extra pounds. And when your children are still fairly young, you've got lots of opportunities to teach them that healthy lifestyle in such a way that they'll retain the lessons well into adulthood.

Meanwhile, you need to keep in mind that your best approach is to help your children develop a strong sense of self-worth and self-respect, teach them about the importance of good nutrition, and help them learn to pay attention to what their bodies are telling them. If they can learn to maintain a sound, healthy attitude to food, and if they feel good about themselves, they're much less likely to fall into self-defeating, self-destructive behaviors like endless dieting and eating disorders.

It's the older child—the child who has reached puberty or the teen years—who'll have the most trouble breaking out of the dieting mindset. This is especially so since this is the age of independence—the time in life when kids begin to declare a degree of separation from parental control and supervision, and are likely to declare that "you just don't *understand!!!*"

Nonetheless, if you approach the subject gently, and with respect for your child's point of view, you may be able to bring the subject out into the open. Remember that this is a time when children are acutely self-conscious, so avoid sounding judgmental or bossy. Instead, be compassionate and focus on creating a dialog.

Once you've opened the doors to communication, you may find yourself tempted to become the disciplinarian—demanding they immediately stop their "foolish" dieting and eat! But keep in mind that the child who initiates such a drastic step is dealing with issues that go a lot deeper than simple weight loss. Bound up in the dieting behavior are confusion, feelings of low self-esteem, fears of being unattractive, fears of not fitting in, and other emotional issues that a simple ban on dieting will not resolve.

Or you may be tempted to go entirely the other way—denying that there's any reason for your child to feel the need to diet. As parents, we rarely want to admit there is anything wrong with our glorious children. They're the joy of our life. Nor do we want to recognize physical traits we would consider revolting. The problem here is that our "unconditional parental love" won't reassure a child who has just spotted a zit on his chin or one who feels bad about her body. In fact, it may come across as a rejection of the validity of their feelings!

The key is to acknowledge how your child feels, and to provide a supportive, sympathetic ear when she is willing to talk about her feelings. Show her you understand, explain how you are there for her and will help her in any way you can. This can be something as simple as agreeing to prepare healthier foods for the two of you—and preferably the whole family—to share, or offering to go for long walks together as she tries to increase her level of daily activity.

Along the way, you'll have opportunities to point out all the good things that go into making her a unique individual. And you'll also discover opportunities to teach her practical lessons about nutrition, health, and exercise that promise better and longer-lasting results than the futility of dieting. In so doing, you'll also be protecting your child from the step that many young dieters take next—dangerous eating disorders like bulimia and anorexia.

That step is taken far too often by young people, particularly girls. I know, because I took a long detour down that road myself. In the next chapter you'll learn all about these dangerous disorders, what you can do to help keep your child safe from them, and what you should do if they've already struck a child in your family.

IF YOU SUSPECT AN EATING DISORDER 10

*U*nfortunately, many health studies have discovered an alarming number of youngsters worry excessively about their weight. More than 50 percent of girls between the ages of 10 and 12 (still in grade school!) express concerns about their weight and appearance, have already been on a diet, and/or routinely characterize food as good vs. bad, allowable vs. fattening, and so on. And girls aren't alone in this dilemma: while girls strive to be ultra thin, boys have their own body-image issues. For boys, the goal is the buff, muscular body of an action hero. And, unfortunately, these attitudes don't begin with adolescence—this concern is also present in very young children. In fact, even children as young as 4 years old are aware of body image—and a few feel that they, too, may not be "measuring up" to the ideal.

These unreasonable concerns are largely the result of the media idealizing these unrealistic images in the advertisements, TV shows, and movies they watch—(and sometimes even from their parents' attitudes about beauty). The American Psychiatric Association estimates that at any given time, a half million people are battling disordered eating.

This number represents only the tip of the iceberg, however, because it's based on a very tight, clinical definition of eating disorders, and focuses on people who are specifically concerned with losing weight. In my experience, dysfunctional eating can be just as bad when it springs from other causes, and the effect can be just as dangerous if it leads to weight *gain* as to weight loss. Thus, my own definition of dysfunctional eating encompasses more than behaviors like anorexia and bulimia, and includes compulsive eating, overeating for emotional reasons, and altering your food consumption for factors other than hunger level (which I'll explain very shortly). Using my definition of dysfunctional eating, the number of people struggling with disordered eating more than triples—and the adults affected by these eating disorders are probably passing their attitudes about food along to their children.

Even more unfortunate is the fact that many medical professionals have no idea how to handle weight issues, particularly in children, and not many health professionals are properly educated to recognize the signs of an eating disorder. That's why it's easy for people to develop dysfunctional relationships with food without anyone noticing!

WHO'S AT RISK

Once an eating disorder develops, it is extremely hard to overcome. It's better to recognize the early warning signs and catch the problem before it takes over your child's life. So, before we explore the clinical definition of the various disorders, let's take a look at some of the warning signs. You've got reason for concern if your child:

- **Eats in secret.** This can mean hiding in their room to eat, or eating away from home often. How can you tell? Check to see if you can find empty food wrappers in your child's room, or their lunchbox or pockets. And if your child is sneaking food at home, you'll start to notice food missing from the pantry, fridge, or kitchen cupboards.

- **Begins skipping family meals.** A child who always has an excuse to be somewhere else at mealtimes, or claims not to be hungry when everybody else is sitting down to a meal, may be trying to hide an eating disorder.

- **Insists on eating (not just meals) in his or her rooms, or insists on eating alone.** Mealtimes are, for most of us, social occasions, so when a child insists on withdrawing from the family to eat alone, this is a signal that something is wrong.

- **Becomes very finicky about food.** While kids do go through periodic food fads, it's a different story when they suddenly start refusing foods that they recently enjoyed—especially if they're rejecting formerly well-liked snack-type foods.

- **Becomes obsessed about foods or particular mealtimes.** For example, your child might begin asking "What's for lunch" while still eating breakfast, or asking if there are "seconds" while still working on the serving on their plate.

- **Spends their entire allowance on food.** This can be tricky to spot, especially if your child is accustomed to having a hefty allowance and doesn't have to account for it. One way to know that this is happening is to notice if they often ask for more money but don't seem to have anything to show for the allowance they've already spent. If you're really concerned, and your school sells junk food, you can question your child's teachers or a cafeteria worker.

- **Seems to turn to food on the slightest excuse.** For example, if your child is looking for something to eat soon after having had a full meal, this is a warning sign of emotional eating. Your child may be turning to food out of sadness or boredom or other, non-hunger reasons.

Each of these behaviors indicates a dysfunctional relationship with food. If you can spot the warning signs, you've got a much better chance of protecting your child's health.

If you believe your child is eating in hiding, approach him or her in a non-judgmental way about why they see the need to sneak food. Perhaps they're worried you would disapprove of their food choices. Maybe they're simply hungry and rebelling against a "no eating between meals" rule. By opening the door to dialog, you allow your child to express his or her feelings—a great way to gently direct him or her away from "emotional" eating.

Skipping family meals is another signal that you can explore without confrontation. For starters, make sure your children know they're expected to be at family mealtimes, whether they're hungry or not. Family meals are a time for everyone to be together to catch up on the day's events—and their day's important, too. This way, attendance isn't a punishment, it's a chance to participate. You can even include your children in the meal preparation. Then they'll be more inclined to attend the meal itself—they'll want to know if their work is appreciated. (And, of course, you'll *love* the salad they made.) And, for the child who insists on eating in his or her room—make it so that your rules simply do not allow it. After all, you *are* the parent.

If your child suddenly becomes finicky or obsessed with food, you'll have to use your better judgement. Most kids go through stages, where they limit the foods they like and cry "YUCK" at everything else. Fortunately, most will also grow out of it, especially if you use the "one-bite rule"—if they agree to take one honest taste of the "yucky" food, you'll allow them to leave the rest.

If your child starts exhibiting any of the warning signs, it's important to take a closer look. But don't rush to judgement! Sometimes events can come up in an adolescent's life that would, in your child's mind, take precedence over spending "family time" at the dinner table. And yes, we all go through phases when our food preferences change. The key is how often this occurs. Is the behavior an exception, or is it becoming the rule in your household? But the bottom line is this: If your child is regularly eating more than necessary—or less, for that matter—there's something wrong. And that almost always means that something is bothering them—feelings about themselves, maybe, or psychological issues that they're having trouble dealing with. So, to help them with their food issues, you need to understand and evaluate these other problems, too!

Take food obsessions, for example. Food obsessions are often hard to handle. Pay attention to what they *do* eat and the circumstances around their eating. Are they only eating the veggies, and playing around with the rest of the food on their plate? Are they taking much longer to finish a meal than they used to? Remember, too, that food obsessions can show themselves not just as compulsions —choosing one or a few foods to the exclusion of all others. They can also show up as avoidances—treating a particular food or group of foods as absolutely untouchable. Pay attention to the way your child relates to food—and *why*. Has he nominated a particular food as a source of comfort? Is she constantly clamoring for it simply because it tastes good or because it has come to mean something more?

The kids who spend their entire allowance on food are clearly putting food above all else, at least in the short term. Cutting off their allowance is not the answer—it will only trigger sneak eating and rebellion. Instead, keep a few sweets available at home (when something's not entirely forbidden, it loses its allure). Or you can open a savings account in your child's name, then make a deal: if they save half their allowance toward some long-term goal *of their choosing*, then they can spend the rest as they wish. (And no fair making it something as boring as college—no young child will think *that's* worth saving for—but you can insist that it's a non-food item.)

AN INSIDER'S LOOK AT EATING DISORDERS

My own awareness of eating disorders stems from something deeper than my professional training. I experienced them first-hand. During my teen years and into my twenties, I discovered the damage they do and the dangers they represent. And I know from personal experience that they can take control of a person's life, and how extremely difficult they are to overcome.

How did it happen to me? Well, you'll recall from the previous chapters that I had lived with obesity throughout my childhood, and that I was put on my first diet at a very early age. For years after that, dieting ruled my life—even though it never worked. In 1978, however, I decided that *something* was going to change. I was tired of the constant teasing I got from classmates and family, I was tired of never being able to wear the popular clothes because they didn't fit me right. I was tired of not fitting in! And 1978 seemed like the perfect time to make a radical change. My family was temporarily moving to a new town that summer. We would be living in the new house for a little over a year before moving into a permanent residence. How perfect. I thought that if I could slim down during that year, I could start a whole new life in our final destination—and no one would have to know that I was ever a fat person!

I started out well. In the first year I lost 40 pounds by eating smaller portions of a healthful diet, skipping snacks, and exercising daily. My family and friends were very proud of me and told me how great I looked at my new weight. The problem is, I didn't see the improvements that they were praising. When I looked in the mirror, all I saw was the same fat person I had always been. To my eyes, there was still a long way to go before my mission was complete—to become a thin person.

By now, though, the weight was getting harder to lose. I became single-minded about cutting my calorie intake even further, and started exercising an extra half-hour every day. That second year was a time of starvation, excessive exercise, and—to speed things up—taking laxatives every once in awhile, all in a desperate effort to lose weight faster. Because I didn't understand physiology, I didn't understand that plateaus—periods when there is no weight loss—were normal. To me they were just another sign of failure. So I reacted to them by cutting calories even further and exercising even more.

My efforts should have paid off by 1980—and to everybody around me, they certainly had. I had lost 43 pounds of body weight, and was now a slim 125 pounds. I was getting compliments from every direction, but I still couldn't see my success. It's hard to explain my blindness, except by an analogy. Let's say you once had a short haircut, but decide to let it grow out long again. You never *really* notice the change in your appearance, because it happens so gradually. But then somebody you haven't seen in awhile comes by to visit—and they're stunned by how different you look now that your hair is longer. *They* can see a big difference, but you really can't see it yourself. Well, that's how I was, when it came to recognizing the change in my appearance after I lost so much weight. I just couldn't *see* it. What I *could* see were the numbers dropping on the scale—and it was like a physical high to see each proof of each pound I lost. It gave me such a rush that I just couldn't quit!

I started talking about my weight-loss frustrations with a close friend at school, and discovered that she was also losing weight. I found this hard to believe, because here I was, living on diet sodas, and there she was, scarfing down a couple of packages of cupcakes! How on earth was she managing *that!?*

She was more than happy to share her secret with me—and that's how I learned about purging. When she told me that she made herself vomit after every meal, my first reaction was disgust. Why in the world would *anyone* want to make themselves throw up? Yuck! But that same night, in my desperation to lose more weight, I gave it a try. Unbelievable! The next morning, the scale showed that I had lost 3 whole pounds!

For most people, it seems unimaginable that anyone would purposely make themselves vomit, but people with eating disorders don't see things the way everybody else does. I was a teenager with a severely damaged sense of self-esteem, and I was desperate not just to lose weight but also to keep from regaining the weight I had already lost. I started getting frantic about calories—how many did my body absorb before I had a chance to vomit them out? I even started getting choosy about the foods I would eat, learning precisely which ones would purge most easily and which ones would not!

After a few months of binging and purging, I managed to lose another 13 pounds in all, and got myself down to a very thin 112 pounds. All of a sudden, the compliments I had been receiving stopped—people were actually telling me that I was TOO thin! By now my perceptions were so skewed that I actually got a boost out of these comments; after a lifetime of being teased as a "fatty," being called "too thin" sounds too good to be true! I became even more determined never to gain back an ounce of the lost weight, and bulimia became a normal part of my life for the remainder of my high-school years, even after I stopped losing pounds. It had become a habit that I couldn't break.

After high school came college, and I became a psychology major at the University of Massachusetts at Amherst. Like all college freshmen, I felt like I was on a great adventure, excited to be moving out of my family home and into a dorm—on my own for the first time in my life.

Of course, my eating disorder came with me—I avoided food during the day and purged after dinner. And I increased my exercise regimen to 2 hours a day. But no matter what I did, I couldn't lose any more weight—all I could do was avoid gaining any of it back. Now I know that this was my body's way of telling me that I couldn't afford to get any thinner, but back then all I could think of was how frustrated I felt. First thing each morning I would plan out my day's food, deciding what to buy after school so that I could binge on it that night. I made almost daily trips to the grocery store to buy cookies, cereals, crackers, frozen dinners—every food imaginable.

By now I knew that something was wrong with me—I was literally throwing money away on food that I'd throw up as soon as I ate it, and I was constantly feeling weak and cranky from the abuse that I was putting my body through. I began to feel guilty and even a little paranoid, worrying that the cashiers would catch on to my eating behavior. So I started frequenting several different markets and making sure that I didn't go to the same stores too often! And although I planned my binges every morning, every night I'd find myself vowing never to do it again.

I felt powerless to stop myself, especially since bingeing wasn't rewarding me with weight loss anymore. So, I simply decided to stop eating altogether. I lived on coffee, diet soda, Bazooka bubble gum, and cigarettes. I didn't let even a leaf of lettuce pass through my lips. Then, in the spring of 1983, it happened. My high school sweetheart decided to come up for a surprise visit. We hadn't seen each other for awhile, and he was absolutely *shocked* at how thin I had become. Out of concern, he spoke to my parents—and they came up to see me the following weekend.

Needless to say, they were horrified at my condition, but they didn't know how to handle it. Dad's solution was to deliver an ultimatum: gain 5 pounds by the end of the semester or he'd make me come home and get counseling. Since my parents were paying for my tuition, I really didn't feel like I had much choice in the matter.

For the first time in my life, I saw that my behavior was affecting more than just me. I was angry with my parents because they were trying to control my life, but I was also ashamed, because I felt that I had disappointed them in a big way. And I was confused and a little resentful, because I didn't see why my choices were any of their business. But I was also afraid—because by this time, even I knew that I had a big problem, but I didn't have any idea how to solve it.

I came out the other side of my bout with eating disorders—anorexia and bulimia—and so can others. But it was hard, because I had lived with the problem so long, and it had become such a huge part of my life. Back then, parents didn't know that much about these terrible conditions, so my own family couldn't help me in the early stages. Half the battle in fighting eating disorders is being able to recognize the early warning signs and intervene before the disorders have a chance to take root.

The mental health community has come up with specific definitions for 4 conditions that fall under the general heading of eating disorders. These are anorexia nervosa, bulimia, binge-eating disorder, and "eating disorder not otherwise specified" (this last category is what I refer to as "dysfunctional eating"). The diagnostic symptoms of each of these are clearly laid out in the "bible" of the mental health profession, the *Diagnostic and Statistical Manual of Mental Disorders*, commonly referred to the *DSM-IV*. Let's take a closer look at each one now.

Anorexia Nervosa

The *DSM-IV* cites 4 specific criteria that indicate a person is suffering from anorexia nervosa. These are:

- Refusal to maintain body weight at or above a minimally normal weight for age and height.

- Intense fear of gaining weight or becoming fat, even though underweight.

- Disturbance in the way in which one's body weight or shape is experienced, undue influence of body weight or shape on self-evaluation, or denial of the seriousness of the current low body weight.

- Amenorrhea. This last criterion, amenorrhea, occurs only in females of menstrual age, and refers to the cessation of menstruation for at least three consecutive cycles, or if her periods occur only after taking estrogen supplements. A related problem, dysmenorrhea, means chronically irregular periods, and can signal that a complete cessation of menstruation is right around the corner. It also refers to girls who fail to begin menstruating even though they are well into the age when they should have started.

The literal translation of *anorexia nervosa* is "a lack of appetite due to nerves"—a vague and misleading description at best. After all, people with anorexia nervosa have not lost their appetites. In fact, they're actually preoccupied with food, thinking about it all the time. They commonly become more interested in food, enjoy feeding others, and are usually very knowledgeable about calories and fat content. Hilde Bruch, a renowned expert in the field of eating disorders, offers a more representative definition of anorexia nervosa. She describes it as "a distinct illness with an outstanding feature: the relentless pursuit of excessive thinness through self-starvation, even unto death."

According to Bruch and other specialists in this field, anorexia usually begins gradually, during the early years of adolescence. It starts off deceptively "normal"—the young person usually simply begins watching their weight or dieting. But eventually, this "normal" goal gets deeply imbedded within an intense fear of becoming fat. This fear, coupled with certain personality traits, can go well beyond simple weight loss.

Victims of anorexia nervosa often share certain personality traits, including compulsiveness, perfectionism, and a feeling that life is out of her control. She is typically female and often believes her life is directed by other people. The only thing she has control over is her own body. In fact, this belief and need for control often initiates the switch from simple weight-watching into a full-blown obsession. She may also be very ambivalent about the changes her body is going through during puberty, seeing her maturing body as a sign that she is growing up and will soon have to let go of the safety of childhood, when she could count on her parents to protect her. At this age, kids often rebel against their parents' authority, but deep down still crave the security that childhood represents.

Once she has started down the road to anorexia, her self-discipline and capacity for self denial drive her to extremes: the more food she avoids, the more "successful" she feels. And even the suffering—the chronic hunger—helps her feel better about herself. Every hunger pang adds to her sense of mastery and boosts her self-esteem. Each pound lost signifies another achievement, so that losing weight and experiencing hunger becomes her obsession.

But as her weight loss continues, she begins to feel the effects of her self-starvation. At the same time, she loses the ability to see herself objectively. No matter how emaciated she becomes, she sees herself as fat, even when she looks in the mirror. This is partly because the change is so gradual—sure she sees the pounds decrease on the scale, and she notices that her clothes are getting too big, but she doesn't make the connection—she sees these changes only as a sign that her "diet" is working!

Spotting the Danger Signs. So how can you tell if your child is in danger of developing anorexia nervosa? You can tell your child is in danger of developing anorexia nervosa if he or she displays any of the signs appearing in the table on the following page.

Taken individually, many of these symptoms may seem harmless. After all, aren't all teenagers moody? And don't adolescent girls typically have irregular periods, until their cycles become established? What you're looking for, however, is a pattern. If your child is showing 2 or 3 of these symptoms, you have clear cause for concern.

Symptom	Description
significant weight loss	a loss of 15 percent or more signals trouble, unless the weight loss is due to an illness or occurs while under a doctor's care.
distorted body image	an expressed preoccupation with body weight, a compulsive or frequent need to check the scales, an insistence on wearing baggy clothing to hide a "fat" body, even though thin.
frequent self-denigration	a tendency to put themselves down often, and not just in terms of appearance; may criticize their intellectual abilities, personalities, or talents as well.
highly critical of others	criticism often centers on how others look, particularly their body shape and attractiveness.
food rituals	eats mainly veggies, drinks excessive diet soda, coffee, or water, cuts food into tiny pieces, plays with the food on the plate, eats more slowly than usual.
cold intolerance	dresses in inappropriately heavy clothing for the climate, complains of being cold when everyone else is comfortable, fingers, nose, and toes are often cold to the touch.
social isolation	avoids food-related social activities with family and with friends.
intense fear of weight gain	expresses a personal concern, makes frequent negative comments about "fat" people around her, makes overly admiring comments about extremely thin people.
preoccupation with food	talks a lot about the caloric and fat content of the food she sees or is given, always counts calories, develops a sudden fascination with cooking and with the eating habits of others, expresses guilt about eating but also enjoys feeding others.
excessive need to exercise	exercises everyday (usually for at least an hour at a time), compulsively, and expresses anxiety if even one session is missed.
amenorrhea or dysmenorrhea	never seems to need new supplies of sanitary pads or tampons, or doesn't seem to use them as quickly as you would expect.
depression or mood swings	becomes cranky, grouchy, or overly emotional, especially when discussion surrounds food or body image issues; food deprivation commonly triggers depression and a lessened control of the emotions.

The Metabolic Complications. Victims of anorexia nervosa are prone to a number of serious complications. Here's a list of some of the consequences that anorexia can cause:

- excessive loss of lean body mass and subcutaneous fat
- dry, scaly, flaky skin
- carotenemia (a condition that causes yellow pigmentation of the skin, associated with excessive blood-carotene levels and usually associated with excess carotene in the diet. Excess carotene often comes from that low-calorie favorite of dieters: carrots!)
- loss of scalp hair and suppressed growth of fine body hair
- constipation or diarrhea, or a combination of the two
- amenorrhea or dysmenorrhea
- fluid and electrolyte imbalance
- suppressed immune system (one sign of this is frequent colds)
- iron deficiency (anemia)
- bradycardia (slow heart rate)
- low blood pressure
- osteopenia (bone demineralization)
- hypothermia (cold intolerance)
- ulcers

LEFT UNTREATED, ANOREXIA NERVOSA CAN BE FATAL!

Bulimia Nervosa

Bulimia means "ox hunger." This translation reflects the classic symptom of the illness: binge-eating. However, unlike compulsive eaters, the binges are followed by compensatory actions such as self-induced vomiting, excessive exercise, and periodic fasting. Bulimics are also known to abuse laxatives, diuretics, or emetics (medications. such as ipecac syrup, that induce vomiting).

For bulimia nervosa, the *DSM-IV* identifies 5 diagnostic criteria. These (slightly paraphrased) are:

- Recurrent episodes of binge eating, in which the sufferer eats a large amount of food in a single sitting *and* feels that the amount eaten and the ability to stop are out of his or her control

- Self-induced vomiting; misuse of laxatives, diuretics, enemas or medications; fasting; or excessive exercise in an effort to prevent weight gain

- Two binge eating episodes a week for at least 3 months

- Constant and excessive concern over body shape and weight

- The disturbance does not occur exclusively during periods of anorexia nervosa. In other words, they have disturbed body images even when they're not actively starving themselves. (Bulimics often go through periods of avoiding foods, followed by periods of binging and purging, whereas anorexics tend to stick to the food avoidance, psyching themselves out of ever needing to eat. Instead, they drink lots of non-caloric drinks and chew a lot of gum!)

Bulimia doesn't discriminate. Anorexia nervosa predominantly affects young middle- and upper-class white females. Bulimia, on the other hand, strikes every age, race, gender, and socio-economic group. It is also more likely than anorexia to occur in boys, although it's still more commonly found in females. When it does occur in males, the victims are usually athletes who must meet weight requirements to participate in their sport. Males, however, don't tend to see bulimic behavior as part of an eating disorder. Instead, they tend to view it as part of their athletic training —and the practice is often even encouraged by their coaches!

Bulimia usually develops in the late teens or early adulthood. Unlike anorexics, whose weight loss spirals to sometimes shockingly low levels, bulimics tend to be of normal or above normal body weight. Their weight tends to fluctuate, though, because their binges are so erratic and their purges are not always efficient.

Bulimia is very prevalent on college campuses. As a Resident Assistant in a dorm at the University of Massachusetts, I knew of 6 girls out of the 17 on my floor alone who engaged in bulimic behavior. I saw then how variable such behaviors can be: some spent hours every day bingeing and purging, while others only did it once a day or a few times each week. But either way, it isn't uncommon for bulimics to consume over 5,000 calories in a single binge, and no matter how often they binge and purge, it's VERY dangerous!

Eating disorder specialists Susan C. Wooley and Ann Kearney Cooke, authors of "Intensive Treatment of Bulimia and Body Image Disturbance," believe that the transition into adulthood is a key trigger for bulimia. They argue that this is a time when people are faced with many changes, both in their physical chemistry and in their life's circumstances. For example, this is the age when many young people leave home for the first time to go to college, when they get their first real jobs, or begin their first serious romantic relationship. All these changes are accompanied by a lot of stress, and for many this stress is just too tough to handle without an emotional crutch that will help them relieve the strain. For the bulimic, that crutch is food, and a fear that the food will make them fat, leads to bingeing and purging.

An additional difference between bulimics and anorexics has to do with their awareness that they have a problem. Anorexics truly believe they are fat and deny that there's anything wrong in what they're doing to themselves. On the other hand, bulimics are fully aware that they're in trouble with their behavior. They just don't know how to get help, partly because they're embarrassed and ashamed of their behavior, and partly because they're afraid that if they do get help, they'll get fat!

Like anorexia, bulimia often begins with a conventional weight-loss program. In fact, this is usually the path that leads to all forms of eating disorders. According to Frances M. Berg, author of *Afraid to Eat: Children and Teens in Weight Crisis*, as many as 35 percent of so-called "normal dieters develop dysfunctional eating behaviors, and of this number, as many as 15 to 45 percent may progress to anorexia nervosa or bulimia within 4 years." Since the teen years are the time when most people start dieting, and add in the fact that teenagers are less realistic about their appearance, it's no wonder that this is the time when eating disorders are likely to make their first appearance.

Bulimia Danger Signals. Many signs indicate a person is struggling with bulimia, and some mimic the signs of anorexia. The table on the next page contains just a few signs to look for.

It's hard for anyone to rationalize behavior like self-induced vomiting, so bulimics are generally aware that their eating patterns are abnormal. That's why they are careful to hide the signs of their behavior from others. This secretiveness is a red flag, signaling a potentially serious problem. If your child routinely excuses herself

Symptom	Description
excessive eating	eating excessive amounts of food with an apparent lack of control over the eating, often accompanied by periods when food is avoided.
excessive drinking with meals	the fluid makes it easier to purge.
disappearance after eating	a classic symptom; bulimics will disappear into the bathroom without explanation or with some excuse (to take a shower), and if there are people around, the bulimic will often turn up the radio or stereo to cover up the sounds of vomiting and flushing.
abuse of medications	reliance on laxatives, diuretics, or emetics to help purging.
strict dieting	this is often combined with what seems like obsessive exercising. (Sometimes the exercising occurs without the dieting.)
preoccupation with weight	weighs herself often (usually a few times a day).
obvious weight fluctuations	this is partly due to the fact that bingeing is usually erratic, and partly due to the use of inefficient purging methods.
mood swings	often tired and cranky, becomes overly emotional or oversensitive, especially when discussions surround food or body image issues. (This is due to self-starvation and the lethargy that vomiting produces.)
cavities and dental decay	acid in the vomit erodes the enamel of the teeth, causing unusually large numbers of cavities.
frequent sore throats	due to the stomach acid, but also due to the frequent abrasion of fingernails against the back of the throat (when the bulimic forces herself to vomit) and the friction of the vomited food rubbing against the throat as it comes back up.
cracked lips and skin at the corner of the mouth	acid in the vomit damages tissue, also a possible sign of a vitamin B deficiency.
frequent heartburn	stomach acid, lacking food to digest, begins working on the stomach lining.
amenorrhea or dysmenorrhea	

to the bathroom after a meal, she may be inducing vomiting—and you've got real cause for concern. Similarly, if your child seems to have a healthy—even huge—appetite at home, but eats very little when you're dining out, take note! She may feel it would be too difficult to hide her purging when dining away from home, so she limits her food instead.

The Metabolic Complications. Like anorexia, bulimia affects the systems of the body. Unlike anorexia, however, some of the complications of bulimia are much more obvious to spot. Some of these complications are:

- frequent cavities
- loss of hair and nail quality (insufficient nutrients cause hair to become dull and even fall out; nails become dull and weak)
- swollen or infected salivary glands (caused by regurgitated food and by fingernails scratching the throat when the bulimic sticks her fingers down there to induce vomiting)
- scarring on the back of hand (caused by the teeth rubbing on the back of the hand when bulimics stick their fingers down their throats)
- amenorrhea or dysmenorrhea
- electrolyte imbalance (dizziness, dehydration, lightheadedness; over the long term this can lead to cardiac arrest)
- constipation or dehydration (usually due to laxative abuse, but also due to dehydration)
- ulcers (due to the stomach acids working on an empty stomach)
- bone demineralization (due to insufficient calcium intake, often because bulimics avoid dairy, falsely believing that such foods are especially fattening; also due to over-consumption of diet sodas—high in phosphorous—which competes with calcium for absorption within the body)

Binge-Eating Disorder (BED)

Anorexia and bulimia have been recognized for hundreds of years, but they attained broad public awareness when the popular singer, Karen Carpenter, died of complications arising from her long-term battle with anorexia. More recently, revelations that

Princess Di and Jane Fonda struggled with bulimia have brought even more public attention to these disorders. But these two are just the most widely recognized dysfunctional eating behaviors. There are others that are beginning to gain public attention because of their increased presence in our society. In recognition of this, two new categories of eating disorders were officially added to the *DSM-IV* in 1987. The first of these new categories is called binge-eating disorder, or BED.

In BED, the victim binges as a bulimic does, but does not compensate for the excessive intake by purging, so it's not surprising that BED victims are typically obese. In fact, some experts estimate that 30 percent of chronic "weight watchers" or dieters meet the criteria for binge-eating disorder.

But binge-eating disorder doesn't always occur alone. It can occur in conjunction with bulimia, as when the binge eater occasionally purges. Or it can occur with a form of anorexia nervosa that is sometimes referred to as bulimarexia. This is something that I did—alternating back and forth between bulimia and anorexia. What happens here is that you get so tired of making yourself vomit that you decide "why bother eating at all?" But then you get so hungry that you just can't stop from bingeing, and then feel the overwhelming need to make yourself vomit.

Both boys and girls are susceptible to binge-eating behavior, although, once again, females are statistically more likely to become victims of it. This is because females are more likely to fall prey to emotional eating—they're the ones who are more often trained to hide their emotions, so they're more likely to turn to other outlets, like food, for comfort.

Eating Disorder Not Otherwise Specified

The final category of eating disorders is very broad, as it's name implies "eating disorder not otherwise specified" (ED NOS). This category covers a whole host of dysfunctional eating behaviors that are not defined within the formal boundaries of the three we just covered. As you can expect, examples of ED NOS are highly varied. They include:

- not eating all day to "save calories" for a banquet in the evening
- exercising for 2 hours to burn off a piece of cake

- periodic fasts (not religious) to "get a head start" on a weight-loss diet
- binging on a quart of Haagen Das after a stressful day at the office
- consoling oneself on a package of fudge after a relationship break up
- indulging in food fetishes (limiting your diet to particular foods or food categories)

All of these things (except the food fetishes) can seem pretty normal—after all, probably every one of us has done one or more of them at some point in our lives.

The danger is when they become habitual. And sometimes they can become astonishingly obsessive. Exercising, for example. Sounds like a healthy thing, doesn't it? But a person with an eating disorder takes it to extremes. I knew one young woman, in her late teens, who would only eat a skimpy salad for lunch, and then frantically jump rope for a solid two hours afterwards. There was nothing rational about this need to exercise—she would become *very* upset if she had to skip the exercise, convinced that she was going to become "fat and ugly"!

IF YOU SUSPECT AN EATING DISORDER

If you recognize a few of these danger signals in your child's behavior, think before you act. You can't expect to reverse the progress of an eating disorder by simply demanding that he or she start "eating right." In fact, this is usually a sure fire way to shut down communications with your child.

One of the biggest obstacles to overcoming an eating disorder is that the victims are often in denial of their problem. Besides, we all know confrontation triggers resistance. Instead, you must take things slowly. And if you don't feel comfortable approaching your child on your own, by all means seek some guidance.

Here are a few strategies that have proven useful for others dealing with these problems:

1. Choose a time and place to talk to your child, without interruption. It's important that you devote full attention and support to your child right now.

2. Don't accuse. Start the conversation with a straightforward expression of concern, using "I" phrases, such as "I'm worried about your health." Don't use accusatory ("you") statements like "You need to eat." No matter how good your intentions, "you" statements will be taken as accusations.

3. Allow your child to speak without interruption. Don't jump in while she's trying to talk. Children struggling with these disorders are often filled with conflicting emotions. They need to express their feelings completely. If you interrupt, not only will you disrupt their train of thought, they're also likely to close up on you.

4. Don't be judgmental, no matter what! In fact, this is why it's important for you to compose yourself before approaching your child. Doing so may prevent any impulsive actions or words. Your child needs your compassion right now, not your opinions.

5. Your child is likely to deny the problem, and even to become defensive or angry. Understand that this is a common response. Meet it with patience, otherwise the discussion may become a fight.

6. Let your child know you understand how scary this predicament is for them. Be compassionate and offer to help them find outside support. You can even offer to go with them, if that would make it easier.

7. Even if your child doesn't want you to come along to their therapy or support sessions, it's a good idea for you to find a support group of your own. There you can learn more about the illness and draw on the strength and experiences of other parents who are coping with the same problem.

Keep in mind that the mood swings and depression that accompany eating disorders can be devastating to anyone, and particularly so for teenagers. Teens and young adults struggling with eating disorders can even become suicidal. If you fear that your child is nearing this point, don't waste any time: *SEEK HELP IMMEDIATELY!*

PREVALENCE OF DYSFUNCTIONAL EATING IN OUR SOCIETY

By now it should be clear that dysfunctional eating behaviors affect a large portion of our population. They strike people from all walks of life, and cause an untold amount of damage to our health. The trouble is that there is no consistent relationship between dysfunctional eating and a person's role, economic status, or age. Whether 5 or 75, with a serious medical condition or merely a desire to maintain health, the majority of our society suffers from some form of deranged eating. And the sad truth is that most of these individuals don't even realize they have a problem. The food behaviors they practice are so common that they're often considered normal. I see it every day in my practice, when patients excuse their eating behavior with the comment that "everybody else does it."

But Everybody Else Does It

It's true—everybody else *does* seem to be doing it! How many women do you know who take comfort in a quart of ice cream or a big piece of cake after a long, stressful day in the office? How about the college students who skip meals during the day, then indulge in a night of pizzas and beer? Or the executive who overindulges in rich foods and drink at a business banquet, then eats nothing the following day to compensate?

What about the "fitness" fanatic who feels the need to "work off" the calories consumed after each meal, or the model who fills up on salads so she won't be tempted by the homemade lasagna everybody else is being served? Then, the most troubling of all, is the 6-year-old girl who declines potato chips or birthday cake because they are "fattening" and she's "watching her weight." Adults, may be inclined to say "how *cute!*" because she seems so precociously "adult"—but that refusal of cake is a very real sign that this little girl is already internalizing some very negative beliefs about herself and her attractiveness, and it's affecting her relationship with food.

Categorizing food as good or bad, using it for emotional comfort, choosing to eat a small amount of particular nutrients while abstaining from others, engaging in excessive exercise to make up for a binge, or following yet another fad diet are all dysfunctional, unhealthy behaviors. They all overlook the appropriate use of food—as a necessary fuel for your body and your mind.

The Influence of the Home

Kids absorb messages about life, health, and proper behavior from the world around them. They draw from all sources, from parents and peers to the media—and then they internalize a select few from which they create their own beliefs. And this is just as true about food and body image as anything else. But when they're very young, parents are their primary role models, and that's why it's important for you to try to set a good example —in both word and in deed, to help them build a strong sense of self worth.

When the parents are constantly disparaging their own bodies and appearance, children learn to be equally self-critical. And when parents base their own sense of self-esteem on body image, children learn to do the same. In my family, I learned this devastating lesson from my Mom. She struggled with being overweight since childhood, and always felt bad about her body. My Dad, on the other hand, had been a professional athlete during his youth, and idealized the idea of physical perfection.

Dad meant well, no doubt, but on many occasions—often in front of me and my sisters—he would openly make disapproving comments about Mom's weight. As a result, my Mom was constantly trying new weight-loss schemes and fads with, predictably, little or no success. What neither of them noticed was that their children were picking up on these attitudes. In fact, I remember that my first fears of becoming overweight began when I was a very little child—I started drinking diet sodas at the age of 5, and my first conscious attempt at weight loss began soon thereafter!

As a result of my own experiences, and my experience with clients in my practice, I have come to believe that the first line of defense against dysfunctional eating is in the home. The first step parents can take to protect their children from the devastation of eating disorders is to create an environment where their self-esteem and sense of self worth is based on who they are, not what they look like!

THE ROOT CAUSES OF EATING DISORDERS AND DYSFUNCTIONAL EATING

Dysfunctional eating, and the more well-defined eating disorders, are triggered by a number of factors. The most common are emotional: feelings of low self-esteem, poor body image, perfectionist attitudes, stress, and anxiety, and in athletes, the desire to enhance performance. A quick glance at this list clearly shows that the strongest pressure comes from *outside*—from society's glorification of certain idealized physical types (thin women, buff men). Secondary causes feed into and reinforce these initial factors—peer pressure, parental pressure, and, in the case of athletes, pressure from a coach or teacher.

But where do children pick up the ideas that trigger such dysfunctional behavior? My own story, told above, shows you how easily a child can begin to internalize the attitudes of the people they love and idolize. But parental attitudes aren't the only influences operating in a child's world these days, as you learned in our discussion of the media's influence (see Chapter 3). Take a look around. Our culture relentlessly reinforces some pretty negative stereotypes about our bodies and the way we eat—and our kids are soaking up these messages like little sponges!

Let's return to our example of the *Roseanne* TV show. We've already noticed that the (obese) characters are portrayed as low-lifes, with pretty appalling habits and relationships—the message here is pretty obvious. But at the same time, notice that every time something goes wrong for the family, at least one character responds by grabbing something to eat or drink—reinforcing the idea that using food for comfort or as a coping mechanism is normal. And look at what the show portrays as normal food—that family seems to live entirely on macaroni and cheese, pizza, sodas, and beer—and the only veggie ever mentioned is canned creamed corn! Sure, the idea was to show how a low-income family manages to eat, but it ignores the fact that healthy meals are possible even on a limited budget.

BOYS ARE NOT IMMUNE!

Though the concern about eating disorders commonly focuses on girls, boys are not immune. In fact, males account for approximately 10 percent of all eating-disorder victims. Like girls, boys commonly develop eating disorders in adolescence, after a childhood struggle with being overweight. And their disorders are triggered or exacerbated by some of the same pressures—to be accepted, attractive and, basically, to just fit in—that girls face.

There are some differences, though. The social image of perfection for girls is to be very thin, but for boys it's to look like sports and action heroes—big, muscular, and powerful. And their eating disorders tend to reflect this difference. They are likely to obsess on weight training, and instead of turning to diuretics or laxatives, they are more likely to seek out "nutritional supplements" that promise miraculous increases in muscle.

In extreme situations, boys may even use steroids—a dangerous practice that has long been a scandal in the world of wrestling and professional sports. The abuse of steroids can lead to a lot of dangerous physical problems, from increased cholesterol levels to liver disease. They can cause heightened aggressiveness and irritability—a condition sometimes referred to as "roid rage." In adolescents, they can even lead to a permanent stunting of growth. In addition, steroid use can cause blood clotting, which then can lead to heart attack or stroke.

At least one expert believes that boys are actually more sensitive about body image than girls. British psychiatrist Sebastian Kraemer, in his article "Boys May Be More Sensitive than Girls," published in the December 20, 2000, issue of the *British Medical Journal*, says that males have more physical and psychological problems than females, citing their higher likelihood to suffer from circulatory problems, diabetes, cardiovascular disease, alcoholism, and suicide. And in adolescence, when girls start shooting ahead of boys in terms of maturation and academic performance, boys are more likely to feel inadequate.

The problem for boys, according to Kraemer, is that they are far less likely than girls to ask for help, in part because society tends to teach boys to work things out on their own. They're supposed to be strong, both physically and emotionally. Instead of seeking help, they're encouraged to downplay or ignore symptoms of distress, and this can delay their access to the care they may need.

While I'm not sure I agree entirely with Dr. Kraemer's thesis that boys are more sensitive than girls, I do share his concern that society teaches them to hide their emotions and to ignore their symptoms of distress. Because of society's expectations, they truly are less likely to verbalize their fears and problems, especially when it comes to eating disorders—because "that's a girl's disease."

THE IMPORTANCE OF PREVENTION

Once eating disorders have become established, they are extremely difficult to overcome. They are much too complex for the majority of parents to manage on their own. And even though the largest percentage of sufferers of eating disorders are middle and high school-aged children, few schools have programs that can educate children—or their parents—about them.

Given how challenging eating disorders are to treat, it's obvious the best strategy is to prevent them before they start. Eating Disorders Awareness and Prevention, Inc. (EDAP) is a group of professionals whose main goal is to prevent eating disorders before they get started. They have developed a brochure entitled *Ten Things Parents Can Do to Help Prevent Disordered Eating in Their Children*, which is available direct from the organization's headquarters at 603 Stewart Street, Suite 803, Seattle, WA 98101. Here, slightly adapted, is what they suggest:

**Ten Things Parents Can Do
to Help Prevent Disordered Eating
in Their Children**

1. Avoid negative statements about your own body and eating patterns, or those of your children.
2. Be certain that your children understand that weight gain is a normal and necessary part of development, especially during puberty.
3. Make it a practice taking people, especially females, seriously for what they say, feel, and do, not for how they look.
4. Scrutinize your child's surroundings for things that endorse the cultural ideal of thinness. (This could include something as "innocent" as teen magazines.) And if you find such things, talk about the images they portray.

---

5. Encourage children to ignore body shape as an indicator of anything about personality or value. It is noteworthy that being teased about body shape is associated with "disturbed" body image and distorted eating. (In other words, kids who are teased by their peers are at higher risk of developing poor body-image and low self-esteem.)

6. Help your child develop interests and skills that will lead to success, personal expression, and fulfillment, without emphasis on appearance.

7. Teach children about the dangers of trying to alter body shape through dieting, the value of moderate exercise, and the importance of maintaining a varied, nutritious diet. In teaching about nutritious foods, however, avoid using judgment-laden contrasts, like good vs. bad foods, safe vs. unsafe foods, and low-fat versus fattening foods.

8. Encourage children to be active and to enjoy what their bodies can do, but avoid putting children into a formal exercise program, especially when they're still very young, unless a doctor advises it as medically necessary.

9. Limit the amount of television your children watch, as well as the number of fashion magazines they read. Occasionally discuss the images of females presented in the media.

10. Refrain from using food as either punishment or reward!!

Francie Berg, author of *Afraid to Eat: Children and Teens in Weight Crisis*, believes that "America's children are afraid to eat. It's an obsession that dims their joy, their curiosity, their energy and their sense of what's normal." If this is true, we must begin our work to overcome this devastating obsession that is ruining our children's health and continues to plague them in adulthood. Our children deserve to feel good about themselves. Childhood is much too precious to be burdened with fears and anxieties. We must show our children unconditional love and understanding. We must let them know they are special just as they are. If we teach them to accept others, regardless of shape, size, and color, we can help them become compassionate and responsible adults—far less likely to fall for the seductive, self-destructive messages that lead to eating disorders.

My Story, A Happy Ending

While it's best to try to keep eating disorders from ever beginning, there's hope even for children who fall victim to them. I know, because I finally conquered my own. Let me share with you my personal happy ending—so that you can see that success *is* possible.

When my family finally realized how terribly thin I had become, they were quick to show their concern. Lacking any other guidance, my Dad fell back on the one thing he thought would work: he insisted that I gain some weight or drop out of school and come home. I finally admitted to myself that something had to change, and I felt terrible that my behavior was hurting not just me but my whole family.

But realizing that something had to change was only the very first step. The problem I faced now was figuring out *how* to make the change. Psychological counseling was out of the question, as far as I was concerned. I refused to have some stranger sitting across the room from me, telling me that they knew how I felt. Like most young people, I was certain that *no one* could understand what I was feeling. Besides, I didn't have a lot of faith in the competence of health professionals. Thanks to the morbidly obese doctor who handed me my first diet book, I was convinced that professional help would just be a waste of time.

I believed that only I could understand what I was going through, and that the only one who could help me was . . . ME! Little by little, I began trying to apply what I had learned from my own experience with weight-loss regimens. I began eating small, healthful meals, and was rewarded by seeing the pounds creep up on the scale. I also signed up for a course in Nutrition, hoping to learn something that I could use to help myself.

One of the first things I did was get rid of my scale. I knew that weighing myself did more harm then good—all it did was provoke feelings of pain and anxiety. I already had enough stress in my life, just trying to handle college and my feelings of guilt for having caused my family so much concern. So, instead of obsessing about the numbers on the scale, I started working on my feelings about myself.

It was hard, especially at first. After all, I'd spent a lifetime basing my self-worth on my weight, and now I had to learn to like myself for who I was, not for how thin I could become. It was a constant struggle to remind myself that I was a worthwhile person, no matter what I weighed.

By the end of the semester, I had gained some weight— enough so that my Dad didn't make me quit school, at least. And although I hated to admit it, I was actually feeling healthier and stronger than I had for a long time. It was still a mental struggle, however—and would remain one for many years to come. All I could do was take each day as it came, and at least my body was now getting stronger.

By the time I graduated from college, I had made a strong re-covery from the worst effects of my bouts with anorexia and bulimia. And that battle had an unexpected, positive effect for me and for my future. I became powerfully interested in nutrition and health, and this interest led me to my present career. As a profes-sional nutrition and wellness consultant, exercise physiologist, and therapist, I've had the opportunity to put my education and expe-rience to good use in helping others to avoid the heartache and physical damage of dysfunctional, disordered eating.

My ultimate victory over eating disorders took a long time— 10 years, in fact—and I had many lapses. No doubt part of the rea-son for this was my refusal to find professional help and support. Back then (in the early 1980s), treatment for eating disorders was still fairly new, and usually involved in-patient psychiatric ther-apy—which I found scary. Today's health care professionals have a much better understanding of these disorders, and treatment op-tions have changed dramatically. You can now receive help and support from a wide range of sources, from nutritionists and med-ical practitioners to mental health counselors and parent or victim support groups.

Part Four

Taking Charge

Nutrition Tips and Strategies

11

It may take some effort on your part to get your kids to appreciate good nutrition, but it can also be lots of fun. That's what this chapter is all about: helping you to find effective ways to introduce healthy eating habits to your children that will last throughout their lifetime.

We'll start with some basics—simple suggestions that will help you improve your selection of foods, along with tips for enhancing the nutritional value of the meals, and even the snacks, that you serve your family. After all, when your shelves are stocked with healthy choices, you can almost guarantee that your growing children will be getting the nutrition they need—even when they "help themselves"!

Laying the Groundwork for Good Nutrition

The foods we grew up eating are the ones we're likely to favor throughout our lives—the ones we associate with the comforts of home and the safety of childhood. By getting your kids used to eating healthy foods early in their lives, you can instill positive habits and preferences that they will carry with them well into adulthood.

That's why I say it's so important to put some thought into your family's nutrition. And your first challenge actually begins when you step through the automatic doors of your local supermarket.

Choosing Wisely

While your goal is to buy the healthiest possible foods for your family, your local supermarket is more concerned with earning the biggest profits they can. And those profits are to be found in the highly processed, pre-packaged products featured in the aisle-front displays and on the eye-level shelves. If you know this in advance, you can avoid the most blatant marketing ploys and keep focused on meeting your family's needs. But it helps to have a clear idea of what it is you're looking for—just what are the healthy alternatives to the heavily advertised, high-profit items?

When it comes to the "staple" items you keep in your kitchen, here's a simple list of choices you can make to pump up the nutritional value of your family's meals:

Processed Choice	Healthier Choice
enriched or converted rice	brown rice, long grain rice
enriched white flour	wheat or rye flour
white bread/rolls	whole grain varieties
pastas made with white flour	whole grain varieties
canned fruits/veggies	fresh, in-season fruits/veggies, or frozen
commercial peanut butter	natural peanut butter or other nut butters
jams or jellies	fruit spread or fruit preserves
canned chili	canned beans you season yourself (kidney, navy, cannolini, black-eyed peas, black)
seasoning salts	fresh and dried herbs and spices
salad dressings	reduced fat version or home-made vinaigrettes
"flavored" crackers	whole wheat crackers, bread sticks and flatbreads

Processed Choice	Healthier Choice
processed cheese food	real cheese
potato chip-like snacks	baked chips, microwave low-fat popcorn, pretzels, rice cakes, nuts and seeds
flavored rice or noodles	brown rice or noodles you season yourself
flavored pasta and pizza sauces	low-fat marinara or canned low sodium crushed tomatoes
sugar coated, flavored cereals	bran, wheat, rice, corn, oat cereals with less than 5g sugar per serving and 3+g fiber (you can add fruit and nuts)
canned condensed soups	low-sodium broth-based varieties
tuna in oil	tuna in spring water (dolphin-friendly varieties)
sugary or cream filled cookies or snack cakes	animal crackers, ginger snaps, graham crackers, shortbread, vanilla wafers

Iodized salt is okay but Kosher salt is more potent so you'll use less. And here's something you might find surprising: honey is *not* more nutritious than regular granulated sugar! In fact, it can be harmful to small children because it can cause food-borne illness (especially raw honey).

Don't reach for the box of "instant" mashed potatoes. It's simple enough to boil and mash a few real potatoes yourself, and it's much more nutritious—not to mention a heck of a lot cheaper! And when it comes to breakfast foods, skip the sugary, brightly dyed ones, with cartoon characters on the box. Go with plain corn, rice, or wheat flakes or squares, then "dress them up" with slices of fresh fruit.

The point is to choose foods in their least-processed state, and to shy away from their highly refined, processed, pre-seasoned, or pre-sweetened variants. You can add your own seasonings or sweeteners at home—and that way you have some control over the fat, sugar, sodium, and additive content in your family's food.

Learning about Labeling

While we're still in the supermarket, let's take a look at one of the best tools you have available to you when you're trying to make healthy choices: the nutrition label that appears on almost all packaged foods.

Once you get beyond all of the eye-catching colors, phrases and glitzy bells and whistles on food packages, you can use the information on the labels to gain better control over your family's nutrition. It used to be that food manufacturers were pretty irresponsible with their labels—they'd say pretty much anything to get you to buy their product. Then the FDA stepped in and established standard meanings for a lot of the more commonly used terms on food packaging. Here's what those claims *really* mean:

"Natural"	Anything they want it to mean! *Everything* is made from molecules and there is no definition for this term YET
Fat Free	Fewer than .5 grams of fat per serving
Low Fat	3 grams of fat or less per serving
Reduced Fat (or Less Fat)	At least 25% less fat than the "regular" version of that food
"Light" or "Lite"	When referring to fat: If 50% of the "regular" version of the product is from fat, the "Lite" version must contain 50% less fat. If the regular version is less than 50% fat, the fat must be decreased by 50% OR the calories must be reduced by 1/3. When referring to sodium: "Light" means the sodium is decreased by 50%
Lean	For meat, seafood, and poultry, this means the product contains less than 10 g fat, 4.5 g or less of saturated fat, and less than 95 mg cholesterol per the standard reference amount (usually 4 oz)

Cholesterol Free	Less than 2mg cholesterol, and 2g or less saturated fat per serving
Low Cholesterol	20 mg or less cholesterol and 2g or less saturated fat per serving
Reduced or Less Cholesterol	At least 25% less cholesterol, and 2g or less saturated fat per serving
Sodium free	Less than 5 mg sodium per serving
Low sodium	140 mg or less per serving
Very low sodium	35 mg or less per serving
Reduced sodium or Less sodium	At least 25% less per serving than the "regular" version
High fiber	5g or more per serving
Good source of fiber	2.5 to 4.9g per serving
More fiber or "added fiber"	at least 2.5g more per serving than the regular version
"Excellent Source" of a nutrient	contains 20% or more of the daily value (used for protein, vitamins, minerals and fiber)
"Good Source"	contains 10-19% of daily value
"More" or "Added"	10% or more of the daily value has been added to the food

It's interesting to note that nutrient claims are typically not permitted on foods intended specifically for infants and kids less than 2 years of age, with a few exceptions. For example, labels are allowed to describe the percentage of vitamins and minerals in food in relation to the Daily Value; "unsweetened" and "unsalted" are allowed to describe taste; and "sugar free" and "no sugar added" are permitted for dietary supplements only!

That's what the words on the front of the package mean. But there's more to learn on the back or side panel of the package, too. That's where the standardized nutrition label appears. Here's a sample, taken from a popular brand of chip—you might be surprised at what you learn.

Nutrition Facts

Serving Size 1 ounce (28g/about 13 chips)
Servings Per Container 5.5

Amount Per Serving

Calories 140	Calories from Fat 70
	%Daily Value*

Total Fat 8g	**12%**
Saturated Fat 2.5g	**12%**
Monounsaturated Fat 2g	
Polyunsaturated Fat 3.5g	
Cholesterol 0mg	**0%**
Sodium 180mg	**8%**
Total Carbohydrate 16g	**6%**
Dietary Fiber 1g	**4%**
Sugars 0g	
Protein 2g	
Vitamin A 0%	Vitamin C 10%
Calcium 0%	Iron 2%

* Percent Daily Values are based on a 2,000 calorie diet. Your daily values may be higher or lower depending on your calorie needs

	Calories:	2,000	2,500
Total Fat	Less than	65g	80g
Sat Fat	Less than	20g	25g
Cholesterol	Less than	300mg	300mg
Sodium	Less than	2,400mg	2,400mg
Total Carbohydrate		300g	375g
Dietary Fiber		25g	30g

Calories per gram:

Fat 9   •   Carbohydrate 4   •   Protein 4

INGREDIENTS: CHOICE POTATOES COOKED IN VEGETABLE OIL (CONTAINS ONE OF THE FOLLOWING: CORN, COTTONSEED, CORN/COTTONSEED) WITH SALT ADDED. NO PRESERVATIVES ADDED.

First, check to see what the label calls a "normal" serving size. That's what all of the other nutrient information is based on. In our example, a normal serving is just 13 chips—and the chips are *tiny*. Serious snackers know how easy it is to double or triple that amount in a single sitting—which means they're also getting 2 to 3 times the calories, fat, sodium, and preservatives!

Next, check the nutrient list. Here's where you may get some pretty big surprises. First of all, keep in mind that the percentages given are based on a hypothetical human—a 175 pound man on a 2,000 calorie diet. Now, let's look at the numbers.

Let's say that our hypothetical man pours himself a bowl of these chips to have as a snack while watching TV. If he shows a little restraint and doesn't fill the bowl to the brim, he'll still easily end up with a triple serving. The label says a serving provides 140 calories, of which 70 come from fat.

Our poor snacker, then, has just served himself 420 calories —15 percent of all the calories he's supposed to get for the entire day! He's also got 21 grams of fat—a full third of his recommended daily intake, and a whopping 540 mgs of sodium—24 percent of his recommended daily intake! All this, while he's getting exactly no vitamin A or calcium—but at least he's getting a little iron and vitamin C. Now, you wouldn't normally expect your snack foods to be high in vitamins, but think of the bigger picture: our hypothetical snacker has just used up a huge chunk of his daily calories—now he's going to have to find some really nutrient-dense, low-calorie sources to fill his nutritional gaps.

Now look at the ingredients list. According to federal regulations, these must appear in order of their percentage of the total product, from most to least amounts. In our sample, "choice potatoes" comes first. Salt comes at the bottom, but its the last of only three listed ingredients!

However, while we're talking about the ingredient list, be aware that with sugar, manufacturers have caught on to what we dietitians tell our clients! So, instead of using just one sugar source, which would bring sugar up within the first 5 ingredients of most foods, they use 4 or 5 different sugar sources in their products. That's why you'll commonly see a combination of things like brown sugar, high fructose corn syrup, corn syrup, maltodextrin, fructose, and honey listed separately—so that the individual sugars will secretly be scattered in the bottom half of ingredients. If you add them up, though, you'll discover that you have a sugary food source on your hands. The key here is to look at the sugar grams and realize that every gram of sugar has 4 calories. For example, a cereal with 12 grams of sugar will have 48 calories from sugar—or 3 whole teaspoons full!

So, how can you put this information into practical use in your own household? Simple. When you're out food shopping, compare the nutrition labels on similar products. For example, in my local supermarket, the product whose label I used above stands right next to an equally convenient, tasty potato chip, but this has reduced salt. The serving size claimed on its package is much closer to what real people are likely to serve themselves. Of the 2 snack options, this is clearly the healthier choice! Even better, you can march further down the aisle and choose a package of flatbreads, breadsticks, low sodium pretzels, low-fat microwave popcorn, or snack-sized boxes of raisins!

BRINGING THE BOUNTY HOME

Once you've made your way out of the supermarket with a basket of healthful food choices, pat yourself on the back. You're more than halfway there. Now it's time to really 'cook up a storm'. The way you prepare your food can enhance or diminish its nutritional value. And if you've been using mainly processed, "convenience" foods up to now, you may be in for a pleasant surprise when you switch to their more natural versions. Processing tends to leach flavor from foods, and after awhile everything comes to taste the same. That's why the manufacturers put in so much salt, sugar and chemical additives—to return some flavor to their products. But if you've started buying the real thing, you've got a whole new world of flavors to explore.

SPA SECRETS

In my professional work I've sometimes been called upon as a consultant at health spas, helping design healthful, nutritionally sound menus for a clientele that expects high quality dining. But you and your family can enjoy this kind of dining at home, too, if you follow the principles behind spa cuisine.

Before we begin, it helps to understand the philosophy behind spa cuisine. In a nutshell, spa cuisine is food that is very low in fat, cholesterol, sugar, and salt. Portions are carefully controlled, because people often come to a spa in order to follow a calorie-specific meal-plan. As you know by now, I'm no advocate of restrictive diets—but the idea of maintaining careful nutritional balance, using healthy food preparation techniques, and portion control are all important in healthy eating.

Cooking techniques are a very important element of spa cuisine because no matter how carefully the nutrients and portions are controlled—if it doesn't taste good, what's the sense of eating it? The goal is to use techniques that maximize flavor and appearance while minimizing fat, cholesterol, sugar, and salt. Here are some spa tips you can put into use in your own home:

- Use non-stick or cast iron pots and pans for sauteing, stir-frying, broiling and baking, to avoid the need for extra fat.

- Use racks in your oven pans to lift meat up above the pan, to allow the fat to run off (drip down) during cooking.

- Grilling, broiling and baking are always better than frying; again, the goal is to keep from adding fat to the food during cooking.

- Poaching is another good option, and you can use a broth made from stock, diluted fruit juices, or other thin fluids (but no heavy sauces, please!)

- Trim off all visible fat from meat. With poultry, you can either remove skin and gristle before cooking, or you can cook with the skin on and remove it before serving. This will significantly decrease the fat content.

- When cooking gravies, stews, or soups, remove excess fat from the liquids. One easy way to do this is to let the liquid cool in the fridge. The fat will rise to the surface and congeal, making it easy to remove. Or you can use a bulb baster to siphon off the clear fat floating on the top of warm liquids, or float a piece of bread on the top to soak up the fat.

If you're worried that adopting low-fat cooking techniques will make your meals taste bland, you're mistaken. The trick is to use herbs, spices, and other flavor enhancers to really boost the taste. Too often we reach for the salt shaker when a clove of garlic, a touch of cardamom, or a sprinkle of lemon or lime juice would take a ho-hum meal and make it *really* special.

Try it for yourself. Make one meal that consists of *only* unprocessed foods you season yourself. For example, how about roast chicken (skip the supermarket's "seasoning" packets) served with baked sweet potato (not canned), and steamed fresh green beans (again, not canned). Season the bird with a few garlic cloves and a few pineapple slices placed on top, and try adding mandarin orange sections and a sprinkle of almonds to the green beans, and a touch of nutmeg and cinnamon to the sweet potato on your plate (though personally, I prefer my sweet potatoes plain). Then sit back and really *taste* the flavors. You may be amazed to rediscover just how good "back to basics" foods can taste!

If you're particularly trying to cut back on fat and cholesterol in the family diet, here are some basic substitutions you can make to any recipe:

If the recipe calls for	Use this instead
sour cream	non-fat plain yogurt
one egg	two egg whites
oil, butter, margarine	unsweetened applesauce, mashed bananas or pureed prunes (in baked goods). In most other recipes, you can usually decrease the fat it calls for by 50 percent, and still have a tasty meal.
cream or whole milk	2% milk (skim milk may be too watery for some recipes)
cheese	use the reduced fat version. Alternatively, you can typically get away with using half of the recommended amount, then adding a bit of skim milk
cream cheese	reduced fat version (it's actually Neufchatel cheese) or Farmer Cheese

And of course, for things like mayonnaise, milk, cheese, and cream cheese, you can always substitute the low fat versions in place of the regular variety. (I'm not an advocate of fat-free for kids, though.)

To reduce your reliance on salt, experiment with using fresh onion, roasted garlic cloves, sun-dried tomatoes, dry mustard, flavored vinegars, and cooking wines during preparation. And don't forget all of those aromatic spices and herbs: nutmeg, cloves, dill, basil, curry, and chili powder can really dress up the foods they're cooked with. Here's a simple idea to make vegetables *really* tasty: saute or stir fry them in defatted broth. Add some garlic and sun-dried tomatoes, and let the veggies cook until just tender. The veggies will absorb the flavors and aroma of the spices, and there's no added fat!

And here's one more spa-cuisine tip: remember that appearance is extremely important. Brightly colored julienne vegetables are both a beautiful garnish on the plate and a healthy part of the meal. Sliced fruits also add color and flavor, as well as good nutrition.

BEATING THE BETWEEN-MEALS BLAHS

Back to basics isn't just for making your family's formal meals more healthful and nutritious. Snack time is equally transformable. For the snackers in your family, you can keep whole grain crackers, pretzels, baked chips, raisins, and popcorn (skip the "butter flavored" and pre-salted varieties) on hand. In the fridge, keep a container filled with carrots, cherry or grape tomatoes, Kirby cucumbers and celery sticks. Natural peanut butter and canned tuna (in water, not oil) are great for making quick sandwiches. And, of course, keep a bowl of fresh fruit in plain sight on the kitchen counter or dining room table—for some reason, if you keep it in the fridge, it always seems to be forgotten!

FOOD SAFETY

While we're on the subject of planning and preparation, this would be a good time to spend a moment or two on food safety. Most people don't realize it, but kids are much more sensitive to bacteria than adults because they're still growing and their immune systems are immature. This means that they're more susceptible to food-borne illnesses. Most food-borne conditions are mild and are often mistaken for the flu, but others can cause real life-threatening emergencies. Here are some tips for safe food handling, preparation, and storage:

- Make sure meats, poultry, and seafood are cooked thoroughly to kill any possible bacteria. Most meats bought in supermarkets have "safe-handling" labels—read them. In general, though, the rule of thumb is to cook hot foods to a temperature of at least 140 degrees, and to store cold foods below 40 degrees.

- Check—and heed—expiration dates (even condiments have them). And check them in the store *before* buying, as well—some supermarkets don't rotate their stock as often as they should.

- Wash all fruits and veggies before cooking or serving—even the ones with skins and peels. They're often coated with pesticides but washing will assure your family's safety. Be particularly careful with imported produce, because other countries' laws are more lax with regard to the use of contaminants. You don't need to spend money on the overpriced "veggie wash" products on the market—just use a scrub sponge and a steady stream of water.

- Be sure to wash your utensils and cutting knives after you use them on one food before using them again on another, otherwise you run the risk of cross contamination.

- After preparing one food, thoroughly wash all food preparation surfaces, such as counters and cutting boards, before using them again, to reduce the risk of cross- contamination. This is especially important with meat, fish and poultry!

LAYING IT ON THE TABLE

A healthy lifestyle goes beyond simple nutrition and fitness. I am convinced that the family and social aspect of mealtimes are equally as important. Mealtimes are when the family can get together and communicate. Also, when you eat together you're much less likely to indulge in unhealthy food habits, as you would when eating alone. In addition, you're less likely to rush with your food and overeat, because you're enjoying each other's company.

Sadly, however, most families today can't share all of their meals together, but every effort should be made to share at least one meal as a family each day. I can't stress this enough! Family time really matters, whether your kids are little or in their teens. So whether you're all sitting down at the table together, or grabbing a bite as you're headed out the door, try to make each meal family time—however brief. It really *does* make a difference.

Remember my warning back in Chapter 8, that it's a good idea to discourage eating with the TV or radio on, because that takes the focus away from the meal? That's just one step you can take to make mealtime more like family time. In addition, definitely discourage children from taking their meals off to eat in another room. And strongly encourage people to remain at the table until everyone else is finished with their meal. This will help a child who tends to inhale his or her food learn to eat more slowly (an especially good habit for an overweight child to get into) because it's no fun sitting around watching everybody else eat.

Finally, as I also mentioned in Chapter 8, avoid "family style" service—where everyone spoons up their own portions out of a common serving dish. Presenting individual servings on each plate allows you some measure of portion control. That way you can make sure everyone is getting an adequate amount of food and that no one is loading up on just one favorite item.

DEALING WITH THE "PROBLEM MEALS"

Most of us can manage to get the family together for one meal, on most days. But let's face it, with multi-tasking families and kids off at school, it can be tough to take control of breakfast and lunch. First thing in the morning, we're all buzzing around in a rush to get off to work or school, and at lunch time family members are scattered, grabbing a quick bite wherever their day takes them.

It's not impossible to impose a little order on this chaos, however. In this section we'll take a look at these problem mealtimes and see what steps you can take to insure that your kids get the nutrition they need, no matter how busy your household is.

Breaking the Fast

You already know that breakfast is an important chance to fuel up for the demands of the day ahead. It helps keep blood glucose and energy levels more stable throughout the day, and blood glucose is the brain's main energy source. Remember: kids who eat breakfast have better concentration, are more attentive, more creative, perform better on tests, and participate more in class than kids who don't.

And here's a scary-but-true fact: The majority of kids who skip breakfast will not meet their recommended calcium intake for the day! This is when they get—or *should* get—25 to 30 percent of their daily calcium requirement. Cereal with skim milk—or even a simple glass of milk as they're headed out the door—is a main source of calcium for kids, so when they skip breakfast they lose about one-third of all the calcium they're likely to get during the day.

But lots of us have very busy schedules, and breakfast time can sometimes seem the busiest of all. If this is true for you, the most straightforward solution, of course, is to just get everybody up 15 minutes earlier—to *make* time for a decent breakfast without having to rush. And it doesn't have to involve lots of preparation time. But if you've got one of those households that just can't "get it together" in the mornings, there's hope for you, too. The trick is to come up with some quick-and-easy breakfast ideas beforehand.

And I'm not talking about those high-sugar, high-fat "toaster pastries," donuts, or danishes. Here are some conventional—and not so conventional—breakfast-food ideas. With all these alternatives, even the most time-stressed household should be able to come up with a healthy breakfast!

- French toast or waffles (if you're feeling ambitious)
- cold cereal and skim milk, with or without fruit
- oatmeal with raisins (made with skim milk instead of water)
- a slice of cold pizza or a chicken leg from last night's dinner
- a peanut butter and fruit spread, peanut butter and banana, or cream cheese and fruit spread sandwich
- yogurt with a handful of cereal or nuts for crunch
- fruit and cheese
- apple and peanut butter
- fruit and whole grain or corn muffin
- raisin nut bread with cream cheese
- scrambled egg and low-fat cheese on an english muffin
- graham crackers with peanut butter or reduced-fat cream cheese, with or without fruit spread
- bread sticks or flatbreads with cheese, or by themselves with a glass of milk
- tortilla wrap with peanut butter and fruit spread, cheese, a scrambled egg or sandwich meat
- trail mix (dry cereal with raisins, nuts, and pretzels) and a glass of milk

- cottage cheese and fruit
- homemade rice pudding, or rice with skim milk and cinnamon
- a "Smoothie" made with 4 oz skim milk, 4 oz yogurt, ice and some berries or other fruit in a blender

Remember to check the labels on some of these store bought foods, especially the muffins. Store-bought muffins can be a big source of fat and sugar—every ounce usually represents about 100 calories. That means a typical 6-ounce muffin packs a walloping 600 calories! And check the list of ingredients—no sugar of *any* sort should be listed among the top three. Ideally sugar should be less than 20 percent of the calories but remember, if you're picking one with raisins, the sugar content will be higher, so check the actual ingredient list to be sure. To be honest with you, I just make my own, 2 dozen at a time, and put them in the freezer. This way I can use egg whites, instead of whole eggs, unsweetened applesauce or mashed bananas, instead of oil; and add raisins, nuts, or wheat germ to increase the fiber. I also cut the sugar in half because the fruit adds its own sweetness.

Also, whenever possible, encourage fresh fruit instead of fruit juice. Fruit juice lacks the fiber of fruit and causes a much faster and higher spike in blood sugar levels because it is absorbed more quickly. However, if your child just won't eat fruit, offer 4 oz. of fresh-squeezed fruit juice. The pulp provides some of the much needed fiber.

Above all, avoid the brightly colored, really sugary cold cereals, no matter how much your kids clamor for them. The manufacturer has to add a lot of sugar in the processing, in order for the cereal to stay sweet in milk. And if that's not bad enough, once the milk has been poured on, kids routinely reach for the sugar bowl to add even more! If your kids are already hooked on sweet cereals, here's how to gradually wean them away from them. Start mixing the "favorite" cereal with a little of the unsweetened kind: about half and half, to start.

Don't expect an overnight miracle, though—they might still want a little sugar on top at first. Keep the added sugar down to a teaspoon, though. Instead, add sweetness by mixing in some raisins or other fruit, and make it even more appealing by adding chopped nuts. Keep it up for awhile and they'll eventually get used to the new taste.

Just how sugary are those presweetened cereals? Take a look at this comparison (published by the Kelloggs Corporation):

Product	calories	sugar (grams)	sugar (tsps)
Baby Ruth Candy Bar	130	18g	4.5
Butterfinger Candy	130	19g	4.75
Apple Jacks Cereal	120	16g	4
Froot Loops	120	15g	3.75
Marshmallow Blasted Froot Loops	120	16g	4
Rice Krispies	120	3g	.75
Corn Flakes	100	2g	.5
Instant Oatmeal (Regular)	100	0	0

Take a look at that last item: Instant Oatmeal. Keep in mind that this is *NOT* the specialty versions that come in all sorts of flavors. It's the flavoring that pumps up the sugar content, after all. And keep in mind that, along with being no-sugar added, you get a hefty 3 grams of fiber in every serving.

When you look at these products, remember that a single gram of sugar equals 4 calories, and a single teaspoon of sugar equals 16 calories. Now, go back and look at the table again and you'll note something that will probably surprise you: a single, 1-cup serving of the sweetened cereals has nearly the same sugar content as a candy bar! And the sugar accounts for more than half the calories in a serving! But look at the sugar content of the non-sweetened or basic varieties, like Rice Krispies and Corn Flakes and Oatmeal. The sugar is drastically reduced. That means that the calories in the unsweetened cereals are more nutrient dense.

Overcoming School Lunch Blues

When it comes to your child's nutrition, the most difficult meal to plan healthy is the one you rarely see them eat—lunch. You can't always count on the school to pay attention to your child's individual needs, and there are always temptations your child will face, from snack foods in the cafeteria to vending machines full of snack foods and candy. Even if your school doesn't have these, you still have to worry that your kids might be trading their healthy foods for a friend's candy bar. Your first line of defense, of course, is to instill a respect for healthy nutrition early on, and reinforce it everyday. Your job is to make sure your child is provided with a well-balanced, tasty meal from home. The rest is up to them.

But what makes a good school lunch? It should include a protein—say a sandwich made with a couple of slices of turkey breast, lean roast beef, or peanut butter and fruit spread. A fruit is always a good idea, as is a healthful (low-fat, low-sugar) treat. Pretzels, baked chips, oyster crackers, and trail mix are popular with kids. And don't forget a drink—skim milk is my first choice, to help make sure kids are getting the calcium they need (and 2% milk is actually available in those convenient little "juice" boxes, these days, or you can fill a small water bottle or Tupperware container). But if they complain the milk is warm or you're sure they won't drink it in school, pack a bottle of water. (Schools don't typically allow for adequate fluid consumption during the school day because children running to the bathroom would break up the lessons!!!). Since small bottles of water can be costly, buy a few to start, then refill them with filtered tap water or diluted fruit juice—2 ounces juice to 6 ounces water.

The trick is to make school lunches appealing enough to compete with the heavily advertised packaged products that are targeted to kids. You can make your own lunch-kits by packing vegetable sticks (carrots, celery, and zucchini are good for this, as are broccoli florets) along with a container of yogurt dip made from plain yogurt and dehydrated veggie soup mix. Or give them a few crackers and a piece of fruit. Or you can stuff tuna, chicken or egg salad in celery sticks or in a hollowed tomato—or simply pack tuna in Tupperware and send it along with crackers and cherry tomatoes. Consider packing a baggie with crackers and chunks or slices of low-fat cheese, sliced turkey breast, or apple slices and peanut butter. To make sandwiches fun, try filling pita pockets and tacos or create wraps from tortillas. And you don't have to stick with sandwiches: a left-over pork chop, chicken leg, or strips of chicken breast with homemade pasta salad or a roll is fine, too.

When You're Out on the Town

We've already talked about the problem with fast-food restaurants. From excessive fats to "super sizing," it's very hard to come up with a healthful, well-balanced alternative in these places. There are some options, however, that are more healthy than others. For example, many of these places now offer a "side-salad" menu, and they've all introduced grilled chicken-breast alternatives to the beef patties. Still, the chicken is usually in a sandwich bun with high-fat mayonnaise and cheese and there's that inevitable side of French fries. . . . And the sheer temptation for the kids is hard to overcome: they wouldn't even consider ordering a healthy dining alternative in a place like this, especially when the chief allure of fast-food is the greasy fries.

You've got more control in the more traditional, family-oriented restaurants. For one thing, you've got a wait-staff that will talk to you, so you can ask how the food is prepared! (Try getting a fast-food order taker to discuss the preparation of your French fries!) Even in these restaurants, though, you've got to pay attention or you run the risk of falling into high-fat, high-calorie traps. Here are some of the most common ones, and how to steer clear of them:

Huge portion sizes. These days, restaurants seem to go out of their way to overwhelm you with huge portions. The typical restaurant portion is actually at least twice as much as you really need in any meal! This is especially true of the inexpensive pasta, rice, and potato servings but even the meat, chicken, or fish portions are excessive. And remember: fat makes food taste good, so on top of the big portions, you can bet there's also a pretty hefty amount of added fat that you can't see! Then to make matters worse, they tempt you to top it off with a huge dessert!

The good news is that most restaurants *do* offer smaller, kid-sized portions. The bad news is that the "kiddie" menu is often very different from the grown-up selection—hot dogs, hamburgers, personal pizzas, and chicken fingers are typical fare, and these always come with a huge heap of fries. In any case, even if you end up ordering from the adult menu, you can ask for a smaller portion—most restaurants will oblige you, but be forewarned, some may still charge the full menu price. Or you can simply exercise a little discipline: ask for an extra empty plate and move some of the excess from your servings to that. You can always ask the server to immediately put half of it in a "doggie bag" to take home with you. (Better yet, share a meal and each get a broth based soup or salad.)

And about those desserts! Kid-friendly restaurants often use their desserts to draw families in. But after a full meal, who really needs a triple-scoop, banana-boat bonanza? Instead, ask your server if you can get a more sensible single scoop, perhaps topped with real fruit (not the almost-all-sugar toppings that are normally used). Other healthy options include a fruit cup or sorbet (instead of ice cream). Or just tell the kids that dessert is waiting at home (where you can control the size of the portions). And if you really want that "death by chocolate" concoction on the menu, at least order it to take home rather than eat it there. That way you can resist the temptation to wolf it down before you've even managed to digest the meal you just ate!

Salad dressing and other high-fat/high-salt condiments. All salads are not created equal. For example, the antipasto offered in Italian restaurants is more like a meal than a salad—every chunk of salami and cheese in it contains 100 calories and of this, more than 50 percent is from fat (it's like getting a teaspoon of oil in every bite!). Then there are the oil-soaked olives and the marinated veggies. Better to go with a green or garden salad instead, but that brings up the problem of salad dressings.

The salad dressing is usually high in fat and sodium, and can contain anywhere from 75 to 100 calories a tablespoon. That's about 400 calories of fat on about 10 calories of lettuce! Restaurants are typically *very* generous in pouring it on—an average dose is 4 tablespoons! What to do? This one's pretty simple: just ask that the dressing be served "on the side." Then you can use it as a dip, rather than drenching the whole salad bowl with it. You may find that your kids prefer it this way—they usually like dipping sauces —but I must admit it can lead to a certain amount of messiness. And don't forget that most restaurants these days offer a low-fat or fat-free variety, or you can skip the creamy dressings and go for the lower-calorie vinaigrette choices.

You can follow a similar "take charge of portion sizes" attitude with other condiments, too. For example, order the baked potato dry and the vegetable side dish steamed, then ask your server to supply butter, margarine, or sour cream *on the side.* This allows you to add just enough to enhance the taste, not drown it. (And note that a typical loaded potato is about 650 calories, whereas the large potato itself is about 250—so again, you're getting 400 extra fat calories.)

It's a little trickier to deal with that ever-present, high-fat condiment, mayonnaise. Anytime you order a tuna-fish salad, egg salad, or chicken salad sandwich, you're likely to get tons of mayo —ratcheting up the fat content dramatically, compared to what you'd get in other sandwich options. Here's an example, comparing two typical SUBWAY 6-inch subs, served without "extra" mayo on the bun:

Turkey Sub	Tuna Sub
calories: 308	calories: 551
calories from fat: 6 grams	calories from fat: 36 grams

What makes the difference? The mayo! In some restaurants you can request that your tuna (or egg or chicken) salad be made with very little mayonnaise, but many (like SUBWAY) can't do that because their salads are all prepared beforehand. Clearly, then, you're better off skipping mayo-based sandwiches in delis and restaurants entirely.

Sauces. Cream- or cheese-based sauces are another problem area—they're extremely high in fat. Far better is to go with broth, or fruit-based sauces, like chutney, peach salsa, and even that old staple of the Chinese restaurant, sweet and sour sauce. A tomato-based sauce is also a good choice, unless it's been made with meat: the fat in the meat tends to cook out into the tomato sauce.

Fried/sauteed foods. Anytime a food is fried—even vegetables—the food acts like a sponge to soak up the cooking oil. Don't believe me? Take a look at this calorie comparison, based on identical portions of fish:

Broiled without Butter	Fried
362 calories (9 fat)	1090 calories (65 fat or 585 calories from fat!)

That's 585 additional calories, all from the fat in which the fish was fried! This same scenario holds true for fried chicken and even for French fries! The culprit is not the actual food product, but the fat in which it was cooked! And its true for those sauteed veggies, too: the vegetables just soak up all the oil from the pan.

What to do? Skip the fried or sauteed offerings on the menu. Instead, go with grilled, broiled or baked fish, meat, or poultry, and steamed or fresh vegetables.

Table munchies. Lots of restaurants put free munchies on the table for you to nibble while you're deciding what to order: nachos in Mexican restaurants, crunchy noodles in Chinese restaurants, the garlic rolls in Italian establishments, and regular bread or rolls just about everyplace else. The problem is that we tend to reach for these unconsciously, and before you know it, the bowl of munchies is empty!

That wouldn't be so bad, except these are usually really high-fat treats. The tortilla chips aren't that bad on their own, though they do contain oil, but there's that guacamole or cheese to dip them in! (If you must have the chips, salsa is a much healthier way to go.) Those Chinese noodles are crunchy because they're *fried!* And the bread or rolls always comes with butter or margarine. In Italian restaurants it's usually garlic bread, which means the butter or oil is already in there, or they serve fresh Italian bread with an aromatic dipping oil to soak your bread in. Why not just cut open the arteries and pour the fat right in!

Your best bet is to just ask the server to take the munchies away—after all, you didn't come to the restaurant to fill up on the pre-dinner snacks, did you? If everybody wants just a *little* nibble, have everybody take just one and send the extras away! As for the tortilla chips, if you've just got to have them, take a couple and opt for the salsa as the dipping sauce—you can have as much salsa as you like! (I even use it on salads).

If you're unsure if a pre-dinner treat (or even your dinner itself) has oil or fat in it, try the "fat test." Just take a napkin and lightly press it on the food. If the napkin comes back shiny or greasy looking, guess what!!!? You've got fat. Food that looks shiny or has translucent bubbles also has fat. And then there's the "mouth feel" test: if it has a slimy feel to it, in your mouth or on your palate, it has fat!

To sum up, here are the basic points to keep in mind when you're dining out with the kids and you want to keep your healthy-living principles intact:

- Take charge of portion sizes. If the servings seem huge, ask for a reduced portion or request that part of the meal be put in a doggie bag and take it home.

- Order the extra stuff "on the side." You can ask that everything from salad dressing to butter and sour cream be brought in separate containers rather than slathered on your food in the kitchen. You can even do this with the sauce that is normally served on the entree itself. All you have to do is ask your server!

- Avoid fried anything: choose soft tortillas over hard tacos, plain black beans over refried beans, brown or white rice over fried rice, steamed dumplings over egg rolls. In Italian restaurants, avoid anything called "fritto" (fried) and in Chinese restaurants skip the tempura (also fried).

- Skip high-fat options: choose salsa over guacamole; avoid anything that's made "con queso" ("cheese" in Spanish). Skip the cheese filled lasagne, canneloni, ravioli, and manicotti, or at least ask for a smaller portion of them. Avoid entrees made "parmigiana" style. These contain a double whammy: not only do they contain a lot of cheese, but the veal, eggplant, or chicken portion is also fried. And steer clear of entrees served with alfredo sauce—this is also cheese based, and in restaurants the cheese is the "real thing," not the reduced fat variety. And remember that certain veggies (onions, zucchini and eggplant in particular) can soak up huge amounts of oil.

- Stick with broth, tomato, fruit, or veggie-based sauces: sweet and sour, marinara, and wine-based sauces are fine. That means you can go with kid-pleasers like spaghetti (but avoid the meat-based sauces) and, for the more adventurous child, chicken marsala or chicken cacciatore. Similarly, kids usually like sweet-and-sour anything, and salsa (although the younger ones will usually want it in its mildest form).

Oh, and by the way—don't worry about those fortune cookies. Each one is only about 20 calories.

KEEPING MEALS KID-FRIENDLY

In a way, the first few months of a child's life are nutritional "no-brainers." It's either breast or bottle, and as long as they're making the appropriate progress in weight and development, you can relax. It's only when you start adding solid foods that things can get a little tricky.

For the Really Young Ones

Really young children are typically more interested in exploring their new environment than they are in eating. They've just discovered that their fingers and toes really belong to *them*, and that they can be used to move stuff around. So mealtimes can get pretty messy—and lots of times it seems as if more food goes *on* little kids, rather than *into* them. What to do?

Start slowly—introduce small amounts of foods, one new food at a time. And keep things bland. Little kids are just learning about foods and tastes and prefer their meals to be bland or only mildly flavored. They also like things best when they're served at room temperature—like Goldilocks, they don't like food that's too hot or too cold. And since they're still pretty much toothless, they're not interested in doing lots of chewing.

To be honest, this early preference for bland foods is something you can use to your advantage when you're trying to raise your kids to prefer healthy food options. At this early age they'll happily accept unsweetened cereals, unsalted crackers, and unflavored milk. So don't sabotage your own goals by trying to "jazz up" foods with sugar—the earlier a kid learns to crave sweets, the harder it will be to break free of the craving later on in life.

Adding Variety . . . A Little at a Time

The first solid food a child gets is usually a specially formulated, rice-based cereal mixed with a little water or formula. As your child gets a bit older, you can start adding a little variety to mealtimes. Try some relatively bland, pureed fruits and vegetables —if you've got a blender, you can make your own and skip the preservatives that the manufactured versions often include to prolong shelf life.

As kids begin to grow their teeth, you can start expanding their "texture horizons." Try offering cut up fruit, cheese, or crackers. Since little kids really like messy eating, try offering these with a "dip" made of pureed sweet potatoes, fruit-flavored yogurt, or cottage cheese. Make sure that the chunks you serve are big enough for their little hands to hold, but small enough to prevent choking. And keep a watchful eye on these early explorations into solid foods—just in case. With little kids, things can happen in the blink of an eye!

Remember not to rush things. It's best to add new foods one at a time, preferably at the start of the meal, when a child is feeling hungriest. And be sure to have an established "favorite" on hand, in case the new food doesn't go over well at first. Also, be flexible: if your child rejects a new food served in one form, try presenting it differently—in a soup, perhaps, or with rice.

Strategies for the Picky Eater

Kids of all ages can go through phases of pretty picky eating. Many parents get caught up in these mini-dramas and turn meal-times into a contest of wills. Don't let that happen in your house-hold! Getting into a mealtime confrontation is a losing proposition for both of you—your child's nutrition suffers and mealtimes become extremely stressful for everybody at the table. Instead, try some of these strategies for success:

- Try a little reverse psychology by designating the contested food as "only for grown-ups." That will often pique a child's interest and make them want to try it.

- Offer the food cut up in fun shapes or decorated in an interest-ing way. For example, if you're trying to get your child to eat more fruit, try topping a (well-established) breakfast cereal with a smiley-face made of a peach-slice mouth and berry eyes. Or build a broccoli-floret forest on your child's plate, complete with mashed sweet potato mountains for dip.

- Use child-sized tableware. Kids can be overwhelmed by bowls, dishes, and silverware that were made to fit adults. Sometimes, just switching to kid-sized versions can make all the difference in a child's attitude toward mealtimes.

- Invite your child to help you prepare the meal. Kids are much more likely to try a new food if they've had a hand in making it.

This last strategy is a good one for another reason, as well. Involving children in the preparation process gives you the opportunity to teach them about sound nutrition. Even the littlest child can help wash the vegetables for the salad—give them a plastic basin with an inch or two of water and let them splash away! (You can always re-wash them later, if need be.) Kids can help build sandwiches, and might really enjoy decorating the burgers with pickle eyes and a ketchup mouth. All the while, you can explain how these good, fresh foods help build strong bodies. While peeling potatoes, for example, you can talk about how they'll provide energy for running and playing. While pouring milk, you can talk about how it builds strong teeth and bones. And so on.

Remember: kids appetites and taste buds are typically inconsistent for the first 10 years of their life, so no matter what you do, you're likely to run into at least a few picky-eating stages at some point. One day your child may want 2 helpings of cereal, the next day it's a struggle to get them to take a few spoonfuls. Don't worry! Although nutrition guidelines talk about *daily* intake, it's more realistic to pay attention to what your child eats over the course of a week or two.

SPECIAL NUTRITIONAL ISSUES FOR VEGETARIANS

Vegetarianism in various forms—ovo-lacto, strict vegan, or other variations on the theme—has rapidly grown in popularity since the 1960s and 1970s. People become vegetarians for any number of reasons, from health consciousness to a commitment to philosophical principle. But whatever the reason for choosing this lifestyle, vegetarianism presents a challenge when it comes to getting enough of the essential nutrients in the diet, especially when it comes to nourishing our growing children.

Now, don't get me wrong—the challenges are not insurmountable. In fact, there are a number of benefits to a vegetarian diet. It's just that, when it comes to children, vegetarians have to pay close attention to the content of their diet, particularly when it comes to getting enough calories, protein, and certain other nutrients to fuel the body and foster good growth and development.

For example, you learned earlier that plant proteins are only 85 percent digestible, so right off the bat this tells you that a vegetarian child's protein intake must be slightly higher than his or her carnivorous counterpart. You can overcome this obstacle if you allow egg and dairy into your diet. You also learned that vitamin B12 is only available in animal products, so if your household is strict vegan, you definitely need to make sure that you're getting this important nutrient, at least by means of fortified cereals, meat analogs, fortified soy or rice milk and quite possibly, a B12 supplement.

The most crucial time to assure a child is getting adequate B12 is when weaning them from the breast to food. For one thing, if Mom is deficient in B12, her breast milk may also be deficient. Also, the bulkiness of a vegetarian diet makes it harder to assure a child eats enough—they'll fill up faster. It's better to avoid complete veganism in the early childhood years. Instead, opt for lacto ovo and add dairy and eggs.

Getting enough calories is also a problem, again due to the bulkiness of complex carbohydrates, the main staple in vegetarian diets. A child may not be able to eat as many calories as needed for adequate growth. This is especially true for toddlers and pre-schoolers. To overcome this obstacle, it's a good idea to include a few servings of nuts and nut butters and to use adequate vegetable oil in the preparation of food.

Most of this is not difficult to do if you are lacto ovo and include eggs and dairy, but it is extremely difficult to do if you are vegan and shun animal products completely. For vegans it's vital to include 1 or 2 servings of fortified cereal, fortified meat analogs and fortified soy or rice milk products into their daily diet.

You'll also want to make sure your family is getting enough vitamin B2, and niacin—all of which are most plentiful in animal products but are available from other sources. The important thing is to make certain that you are getting adequate amounts of these vitamins from alternative—that is, non-meat—sources. Getting enough calcium, iron and zinc can be tricky, too.

Remember: although the iron content of a vegetarian diet can be high, the iron is in the less absorbed non-heme form. The good thing is that vitamin C has a strong presence in vegetarian diets —as you'll recall, vitamin C helps the body absorb iron. Calcium, on the other hand, is usually not a problem for lacto ovo vegetarians, but it is for vegans. The trick is to assure adequate intake of calcium-fortified soy or rice milk and fortified meat analogs.

One way to insure that your kids are getting all the nutrients they need in a vegetarian household is to serve "fortified" alternatives.

For example, if you've eliminated dairy from your diet, opting for rice or soy milk instead, make sure that the brand you buy is fortified with calcium.

And here's a special concern for vegans who live in the northerly regions: watch out for a vitamin D deficiency! You'll remember from the discussion earlier that a vitamin D deficiency is particularly damaging to bones—the long bones of the legs can become bowed, and the bones of the skull can become soft. Generally speaking, our primary dietary source of vitamin D is in fortified milk, but you'll remember that this is the one vitamin our bodies can make for themselves—from sunlight. For people who don't live in the sunny south, getting enough exposure to sunlight in the winter months can be tough. Once again, the answer is to make sure your rice or soy milk-substitute is fortified with this important vitamin, too.

So, what are the basic elements of a healthy vegetarian diet? First, make sure the diet is calorie dense and supplies enough energy for adequate growth. Next, make sure that each meal contains a healthy serving of fruits, vegetables, whole grains, and legumes. At least 2 servings of nut butters, nuts, seeds and fortified tofu or meat analogs should be consumed daily, along with 2 to 3 servings of fortified dairy, soy, or rice milk—be sure the label says its fortified to 25 percent of the daily value. You also need to make certain that you occasionally (a few times per week) include plant oils and/or eggs. And keep an eye on water intake—six 8-ounce glasses per day is the absolute minimum.

For vegetarians who need help in making sure that their families are getting enough of the essential nutrients in their diet, there are a number of resources available, especially on the Internet. Three good sites, where you can find specially tailored Vegetarian Food Pyramids and plenty of guidance, are offered at www.vrg.org, a site sponsored by the Vegetarian Resource Group, and at www.oldwayspt.org and www.vegsource.com.

FITNESS FOR THE FAMILY

12

I've said it before and I'll say it again: a design for a healthy lifestyle is not complete if it doesn't include physical fitness. But I'm not just talking about jumping jacks, leg lifts and push-ups—unless that's what works for you, of course. Instead, I'm talking about building physical activity into your everyday life. This is especially important for our kids, for far too many children spend way too much time in sedentary pursuits: watching TV, playing video games, or "surfin' the 'net."

But how do you motivate a junior couch-potato to get active? In this chapter I'll share with you some ideas that I've found helpful, both in my practice and in my efforts to keep my own child healthy, active, and fit!

GETTING INTO THE FITNESS HABIT

The good news is that, once you get kids going, they're likely to *keep* going. Most little kids are like nature's own *Energizer Bunnies*—they can keep going, and going, and going. Of course, the longer a child has had to develop sedentary habits, the harder it will be to reverse the trend, but it's never impossible. The trick is to work with what you've got and maximize the opportunities for your child to get active. Remember—everyday activities are just as valid forms of exercise as anything you might do in a gym!

Everyday Exercise

When children are old enough to walk, let them walk! Don't carry them just because you're in a hurry. And don't opt for the stroller every time you go out. It's appalling how often parents pop kids—even pretty big kids—into strollers. Sure, little kids have short legs, so they'll slow you down when you're in a rush, but that's no excuse for turning them into passive, full-time passengers. We need to have more patience, so that our children learn how to do things for themselves! Match your pace to theirs. And who knows, their slower pace may be just what you need to slow *yourself* down and reduce your own stress.

On the other hand, if your child is just bubbling with energy, you can use the opportunity to step up the activity a little while still keeping it fun. They might like to get into a walking, skipping, or hopping "race" with you. They'll love the attention (especially if they get to "win"), and they'll be getting lots of good exercise without realizing it, not to mention positive reinforcement for their achievement when they "beat" you. And there's another benefit to such games. When they see you taking your "losses" with good grace, it helps them to learn about how to be good sports.

And while we're on the subject of setting an example, remember that you're the most important role model in your child's life. You have lots of opportunities to set an example for them, both subtly and directly. If you appreciate the benefits of physical activity, some of that attitude *will* rub off on your kids. Talk about how great it is to be able to move freely, and about how life would be so very different if we didn't have that freedom to move. And above all, be active with them!

The great thing about these informal, everyday activities is that they put very little performance pressure on children. As long as you don't make a big deal about how fast they go (except when praising their lightning speed, that is) or how hard they try, they won't develop performance anxiety or a fear of failure. They'll be more interested in the sheer pleasure of activity, instead of worrying about living up to your expectations. And while it's great to talk about how good it feels after being active, don't focus on the weight-loss or body-building aspect of it. Focus on the rejuvenating energy you get from it! You want them to enjoy exercise for its own sake, not to obsess over it.

The Great Outdoors

If the weather is good and you live in a community where the kids are safe playing outdoors, sometimes it's enough just to banish them from the house for a while—once outside, they're bound to find something to do that requires movement. My son gets *tons* of exercise just running around in the backyard, playing with the dog! Riding trikes or, for older kids, bikes or rollerblading, are other fun activities that even the most exercise-phobic kids won't consider as being "exercise."

If you live in a cold climate, winter brings even more opportunities: cross-country skiing, ice skating, and snow-shoeing are the obvious ones, but there's a lot of activity involved in sledding and in building snowmen or snow forts too! And a good snowball fight can get even the least active kids into the spirit of movement. In fact, just walking in deep snow counts as vigorous activity—and young kids just *love* being the first to leave footprints in a deep patch of freshly fallen snow.

It helps to keep a good supply of active games on hand to encourage your children to play. If you've got a yard, set up a volleyball net in spring and keep the equipment handy—the kids will play all summer long. Just keeping a few balls around will yield lots of different activities, too—a softball, some tennis balls, and a basketball can be used in all sorts of games. Games like catch and dodgeball are great for groups, but a solitary session of dribbling a ball down the driveway, or just tossing it against the house and chasing it when it bounces back can burn up a lot of energy too! And there are lots of active games that don't need any equipment at all. Games like *Red Rover* or *Mother May I, Tag,* and *Red Light-Green Light* are great when there's enough kids around.

If your neighborhood doesn't provide opportunities for active play—if you live in a heavily built up urban area, for example—you can always make use of the public areas in your community: most cities have parks, skating rinks (ice or roller), and playgrounds that are open to the public. Or check out local hiking trails. Make it an expedition, with a picnic lunch if the weather is nice, or a thermos of hot cocoa to share in winter.

And remember, as much as we want to protect our children from harm, it's healthy to accept the fact that they'll inevitably pick up a few scrapes, skinned knees, and other "boo-boos"—it's all a part of being a kid. Within reasonable limits, we must encourage our children to test their physical limits and avoid being too restrictive. Tree-climbing and rollerblading, while they may give the overprotective parents among us a little hesitation, can give older kids a great workout, as long as they're developmentally ready for it.

Bringing Exercise Indoors

If your kids don't have access to the "great outdoors" but you have enough space—say a basement, patio, or spare room—make space for the kids to rollerskate, ride scooters and trikes, and run around in there. You can lay a couple of exercise mats or thick comforters on the floor, set up a boom box, and encourage the kids to use the space for tumbling, calisthenics or just silly play. If your space is more limited, don't despair—there are lots of creative ways to bring active living indoors.

For example, a game like *Twister* takes only a small patch of clear floor, but can give a handful of kids a lot of squirming activity. Or turn up the radio and get the kids dancing! Little ones will be thrilled to dance with you, although by the time adolescence approaches you'll probably have to relinquish the floor. Daughters in particular seem to find it agonizingly "uncool" to think their parents would even *try* to do the current steps, and the ones you recall from your own teen years will seem hopelessly out of date, no matter *how* smooth you think you are.

Make the kids' rooms activity friendly. For younger children, a thick mat instead of a lightweight floor covering will provide a place for exercising, while protecting knees and elbows from the hard floor. For older children, pop a chin-up bar in the doorway—it will get a workout, particularly by teenage boys. A pair of exercise bands are a good idea, too.

And don't forget that household chores also count as exercise. During chore time, turn up the radio and get everybody dancing while they work! Not only are you all getting fit, the chores will seem less boring, too.

Keeping Things Positive

No matter what activities you encourage your child to get involved in, the important thing is to keep them fun and stress-free. This is especially critical when children are overweight or feel unsure of their athletic abilities. Many children enjoy group activities involving other children, and these are good for building their sense of teamwork, but an overweight child who feels clumsy or is self-conscious about how his or her body looks can find such group activities embarrassing and humiliating, so never force the issue.

And while you want to celebrate a child's achievements and give positive reinforcement as often as you can, don't stress success in such a way that your child feels like a failure if he or she misses a goal or drops the ball. Cheer the effort, not just the success! Remember, your goal is to make being active fun and rewarding so that your child will want to make it a regular habit, one that will last a lifetime.

IT'S ACADEMIC

Unfortunately, many of us can't count on our schools to reinforce the fitness message, in part because many schools have cut their regular physical education curriculum. Furthermore, safety concerns have even eliminated outdoor recess periods in many communities. This is particularly detrimental to our children's health because schools provide the perfect physical and social set-up for active play. Most schools have adequate space, and there are always enough kids gathered together to make a team for any sport or game that strikes their fancy. Even better, unlike in community-based sports, the kids in a class or grade already know each other well enough to work together on a team.

But even if your child's school doesn't have a formal physical education program, many school boards are open to requests to put the facilities to use. You might want to try to get enough other interested parents together and petition for the use of the school's playing field or gym. If you've got volunteers to coach and chaperone the kids, you'll make it pretty hard for the board to say no. (And even if they *do* refuse your request, you'll have formed an interested group with whom you can organize your own activities, off school property, if need be.)

DO-IT-YOURSELF FITNESS, IN STAGES

As you can see, there are many creative ways to bring activity into your child's life. But keep in mind, exercise is not a "one size fits all" enterprise. As you learned in Chapter 6, activities need to be kept developmentally age-appropriate. Here are some ideas that will help you work up a fitness plan no matter what stage your child is in.

Fitness for Infants

Healthy infants who are fed a reasonable amount, are not overfed, and are growing at a consistent, standard rate do not need anything special in terms of fitness or exercise. More important, at this stage in life, is that they are encouraged in their own natural development process, and given every opportunity to be nurtured, bond with their parents or caretakers, and explore their surroundings.

In addition, it's important that babies be dressed loosely enough to allow them to move their limbs freely. This is especially important as they grow stronger and more capable of controlling their movements. You can make a game of letting them push their feet or hands against the slight resistance of your hands or against your lap. It gives them a chance to use their muscles without risking undue stress on their little limbs. When they're ready to start trying to crawl, it's a good idea to provide a safe place to practice, like a mat or blanket on a clean floor, so there's no danger of falling.

Once a child is able to crawl, you can work with them to encourage learning about and experiencing their surroundings. In the beginning the crawling is awkward but soon you'll be amazed at how quickly those little buggers can cruise around the living room. Before long your youngster is making an all out effort to walk—latching on to tables and couches, in an attempt to boost themselves up on their feet. And the next thing you know, they're running down the hall.

Keep in mind that every child is different. There are some who crawl for what seems like an eternity, getting where they want to go faster than a bolt of lightening on their hand and knees, while others seem to almost skip the crawling phase and go straight to walking and running. But whatever phase your little one is in, remember that all this movement counts as healthy activity! And it's funny: when they're born, we can't wait for them to crawl; when they crawl, we want them to walk—but then once they walk, which quickly turns into a run, we wish they would just sit still sometimes!

Finally, remember that babies—especially the very youngest ones—do a lot of their growing and developing during their sleep. That means it's important to provide a safe, comfortable sleeping place, preferably some place specifically dedicated to "bed-time," like a crib or cradle. The actual amount of sleep a baby needs each day will vary, as naps and activity levels vary, so I can't offer you a single "target" amount of sleep. But typically a young child needs anywhere from 10 to 12 hours a day. If you're concerned that your child isn't getting enough sleep, consult your pediatrician.

For the Toddler and Preschool Set

Little kids are simply *not* going to be interested in exercise for fitness—all they really care about is having *fun!* They're not going to be stimulated to do anything if it has lots of rules and feels like work. And since kids this age are developing their fine motor skills and have pretty short attention spans, your best bet is to provide lots of variety. You're also going to need to have a sense of humor because things don't usually go exactly as you plan. Kids this age are likely to get excited and act "out of control"—and even go a little goofy on you, but hey, that's what being a kid is all about. If they can't act silly when they're young, when can they?!

What kind of activities keep kids this age interested? Here's a list of some sure-fire options:

- Create a pseudo 'training' circuit with various "stations," each with a different activity. Among the stations, you could include bouncing a ball, building a tower of large plastic blocks, hopping on one foot, punching the air, kangaroo or bunny jumps, and walking on all fours. Keep the activities simple and easy to do.

- Tickling and wrestling games (*gently*). But be sure to pay attention to your child's mood. Sometimes these sorts of games get intense, so if those delighted squeals start sounding a little like breathless moans, your child is not having fun anymore.

- One-on-one games of tag or catch with Mom or Dad are always a big hit. Little kids really love being the center of a parent's attention, and a parent's praise at this age is a massive self-esteem booster.

- As mentioned earlier, this is a great age for dancing. The sillier the better!

- A rousing session of jumping on the bed—fully supervised, of course! To a kid, there's something deliciously naughty about this, even when Mom or Dad is jumping right beside them!

The important thing when picking activities for a child of this age is to make the activities feel like games, not chores. And you want to keep the activities within your child's skill level. You're not trying to initiate your children into Olympic training, you're trying to help them develop their motor skills and teach them that being active is a fun, happy part of living.

School-Agers

As kids get older, their interests become more focused and individual. You can take advantage of this in your efforts to keep them active. Got a son who loves the water? Swimming, whether on a swim team or just for fun, is great exercise. Got a daughter who's just fascinated by nature? Go hiking and make the event a collectors expedition (if you're lucky, she'll just want to bring home leaves and flowers; but be prepared for a request to bring home additions to her bug collection, if that's where her interests lie).

At this age, kids often begin to enjoy the social aspect of activity, and organized team sports are a good way to guarantee regular exercise along with a healthy exposure to competition, teamwork, and good sportsmanship. Just make sure that you select an organization that places its emphasis where it belongs—on ensuring that all the team members get a chance to play and have fun—instead of on winning at any cost. There's nothing more turn-offish then sitting on the bench watching everyone else play ball!

Fun-for-all family activities are also more enjoyable at this age: bike rides, rollerblading, family ski trips, bowling, and even a day at the beach or the park, complete with a Frisbee, volleyball, touch football, or snorkeling. For the more adventurous, there's hiking and rock-climbing.

Jumping rope, playing hop-scotch, and tag are all age appropriate. You can "play tag" with pre-schoolers, too, but you have to bend the rules a lot—there's nothing more frustrating for a little child than to be "it" and never be able to catch the bigger players.

More formal exercise regimens are possible for school age kids, but they shouldn't be too intense. At this age, elastic exercise bands, tumbling, calisthenics, water aerobics, and working with light 1 to 2 pound weights are all appropriate, if they're what your child enjoys. And you don't even need to buy expensive weights. 16-ounce vegetable cans work just as effectively as one pound dumbbells. If your child is interested in more formal instruction, martial arts classes are a popular option. In many instances you can even sign up to take the classes together!

One thing to keep in mind about kids at this age is that they generally don't have a "sense of pace." They'll typically give their all in a sport or activity, without realizing that they'll eventually poop out. Unfortunately, just before they "hit the wall" of exhaustion, they're likely to lose concentration and are vulnerable to getting hurt. They tend to have no regard for safety when they're caught up in the excitement of an activity, so supervision is really important.

Remember too that this is an age when children really *care* about how the world—and especially their peers—think of them. That makes them very easily hurt, emotionally, if they feel that they don't perform well. This can make them self-conscious, and can make some kids start to turn away from physical activities because they're afraid of looking awkward or just not being "good enough." You can help avoid this by being supportive and by keeping your priorities straight: If you act as if "winning is everything," your child will pick up on it, and any failure to excel will really hurt his or her sense of self-esteem!

Whatever activity your child finds most interesting, make sure to select the proper clothing for it. Loose fitting cotton clothes allow for free movement. It's usually a good idea to dress a little lighter than the temperature calls for, because strenuous activity will raise their body temperature. But in really cold weather have them dress in layers—they can always peel off a layer as their actions warm them up.

Tips for Teens

Teenagers are tricky beasts. Sometimes it seems like they're bound and determined to do exactly the opposite of anything you suggest—even when you *don't* have a classic rebel-child on your hands. This makes encouraging activity a little harder than it is with younger kids, especially if your teenager is new to regular exercise. It helps to remember that, at this age, teens are most attracted to "adult-like" things—they usually respond well to things that feed into their need to be treated like grown-ups. Tailoring your suggestions to this tendency will get you better results than simply nagging them to "get active."

For example, teenage boys often idolize athletes—so suggesting a training program that incorporates muscular endurance and cardiovascular activities, like the one their sports heroes follow, might work well. Many teenage girls, on the other hand, enjoy structured aerobics classes, like that of their female cohorts. Once again, pay attention to your child's individual interests, their abilities, and their personality. Some kids are natural loners, uninterested in group activities, while others are happiest if exercise can also be a social event.

The good news is that, at this age, the physically adept teen does have more options available than younger kids have. By junior high, and especially by high school, there are usually a variety of teams and sports-oriented clubs, that the lower grades simply don't offer—sports like baseball, softball, basketball and track and field, to name a few. On the other hand, there are fewer opportunities for non-athletic kids to get active.

Team sports can be a great outlet for a teen's energy and helps them stay fit, but it's equally important to make sure they're properly coached. Remember, this is a time of accelerated growth, and over-training can lead to long-term damage. A competent coach is aware of these special risks and works to eliminate them. The problem is that high school coaches come with their own set of fallacies about training—this is something you should *definitely* be aware of. For example, back in my old high school I remember one wrestling coach who encouraged his team members to wear plastic suits while running. He believed that this helped them to make weight —achieve the proper weight for their wrestling class. But this is definitely an unsafe training practice and that coach should have known better than to use it. As parents, we need to be aware of such things, and put a stop to them!

At the other extreme are the teens who aren't into the whole "jock" thing. They rarely move unless they have to. The majority of these teens, if they're at a relatively appropriate weight and stick to a predominantly healthy diet, will be able to maintain their weight because they have the luxury of a youthful metabolism that will temporarily compensate for their couch potato lifestyle. My concern, however, is with the long term. It will be much harder for them to adopt a physically active lifestyle once they've become accustomed to a sedentary one. And even though they're at a "normal" weight at the moment, they're certainly not fit! Activity is important for more than just keeping weight down, it's necessary to develop muscles, and a sedentary lifestyle does *nothing* to help in this regard.

And it doesn't help that this is the age of agonizing self-consciousness for lots of kids, and the bodily changes that puberty triggers often doesn't do much for their coordination either. This sometimes makes it hard to get a teenager to try something new in the world of athletics—they're immensely afraid of looking uncool.

Also, keep in mind that kids this age are torn between wanting to be kids without boundaries and being treated as responsible adults. They are extremely careful not to appear "childish" in front of their peers. This can actually work to your benefit, because you can take advantage of their desire to participate in "adult" activities. They like going to the gym to work on the machines or attending structured exercise classes. In addition to aerobics, girls are typically interested in step, yoga, and spinning programs, whereas boys tend to gravitate to anything called "training." This can mean anything from weight machines to martial arts.

If your own lifestyle has led you to be sedentary lately, this can be a great opportunity for you, too. You can sign up for a program *with* your teen, or work out an at-home exercise regimen that you can do together. No more excuses!

THE RELUCTANT ATHLETE

If you've got a reluctant athlete on your hands, what to do? First, don't push. Instead, try a more subtle approach. Make opportunities for exercise and, if your teenager is exceptionally self-conscious, provide some privacy in which to practice, at least at the beginning. This is the age when it's a really good idea to provide exercise opportunities in your child's room—a chin-up bar, a set of elastic exercise bands or light weights, an exercise mat and an exercise video—where they can do their own thing without having to worry about being caught "looking dorky." For a lot of kids, this private practice time will ultimately yield to a sense of mastery, and the fear of being uncoordinated and clumsy will gradually disappear.

Second, provide non-stressful opportunities for activity that don't challenge your teenager's fears of failure. Even non-swimmers can have a lot of fun and get a good deal of exercise at the beach or the pool. To beef up the exercise content of a session in the water, you can buy webbed gloves for more resistance with strokes. For do-it-yourselfers, you can fill one-quart plastic bottles with water to use as weights, and you can use noodles as floats to allow for lower-body calisthenics.

Bicycling and hiking are two other good activities that don't usually challenge a teen's sense of dignity. And in cold weather climates, there's cross-country skiing and snow-shoeing. For the non-athletically inclined, cross country is less intimidating than downhill skiing because the sense of control is greater—and it provides a great full-body workout!

THE INVULNERABILITY COMPLEX

One thing to keep an eye out for, especially if your teen is athletically inclined, is the tendency to overdo it. Teens are notorious for believing that they're invincible—they'll often indulge in risky, excessive, or dangerous behaviors because "bad stuff only happens to other people." So, you can't count on them to use good judgment on their own behalf. Keep this in mind if your teen decides to get involved in weight-training—they may become over-enthusiastic and risk injury by pushing themselves too hard.

The same is true in sports, where they'll push themselves to the extreme. If this happens, try hard not to nag them about it. There's no quicker way to turn a teenager deaf to your advice than to nag. Instead, try engaging your teen in a calm, rational conversation and avoid anything that sounds accusatory. No "you should's" or "you shouldn'ts"—keep the issues objective rather than personal.

MAKE IT A FAMILY AFFAIR

If you've been finding excuses to put off beginning your own exercise program, now would be an ideal time to get started—by exercising with your child. Your own participation in physical activity will set a great example for your child, and even the most independent teenagers look to their parents as role models, though they'll rarely admit it. If you've been lax at exercising and your kids are still quite young, working with them is an excellent way to ease into a more active approach to life—their age-appropriate activities can be your gentle introduction to exercise, and once you've become more accustomed to physical activity you can gradually expand your own exercise options.

CREATING A NEW COMMUNITY

13

*I*n the past couple of chapters we've discussed practical advice for enhancing your family's nutrition and explored ways that can help you inspire your children (and your whole family) to become more active. But when it comes to creating a healthy lifestyle, you can't stop there. There's a whole other area that needs work as well—let's call it "values and community." In this chapter, I hope to help you recognize the important role that these concepts play in your life and, particularly, the life of your child, and to give you sound and practical guidance on how you can work to create the sort of community that will support your child as he or she grows and develops.

WHAT'S SO IMPORTANT ABOUT COMMUNITY?

We all know by now that eating nutritious foods and engaging in daily activity will help us to become healthier. But across the country, today's health professionals are beginning to recognize that there are other, equally important, areas of our lives that also have a powerful impact. In fact, some of the most prestigious medical schools now offer courses in holistic and alternative medicines.

Health professionals are interested in exploring these spiritual and religious based areas because they are beginning to recognize that patients—people—are more than just a collection of body parts; not that they didn't already know that their patients were people, it's just that prior medical training focused on disease and medication. Fortunately, they're now beginning to realize that emotions, attitude, and outlook play a very important role in our general wellness, too. Mental well-being is something I've recognized for a long time, in part because of my experiences as an overweight child and, subsequently as a victim of eating disorders. The emotional element created the base for my disordered eating and was impossible to miss—and once I began working with patients in my clinical practice, I encountered the same issues that I had wrestled with, time and again in my patients.

But emotional health is difficult to achieve and maintain when your environment is a vacuum. We are social beings, and we look to our communities for recognition, acceptance, and support. We take inspiration from the example of others, and we develop our taste, our goals, and often our self-esteem in part from what we see as the values and judgments of others.

Thus, the community in which we live has a profound impact on what we think about ourselves and, as a result, on how we take care of ourselves. Unfortunately, as I discussed in the earliest chapters of this book, our "community" has grown less supportive even though it has grown more expansive. In place of local communities where everyone knew their neighbors, we've got a global community of bodies in which individual people seem to be valued only as "consumers"! No wonder so many of our kids are feeling alienated, stressed-out, and unimportant—and no wonder so many of them are responding to all of these negative feelings by turning to unhealthy relationships with food.

WE DON'T HAVE TO TAKE IT

From industries and advertisers to politicians and social policy, it can seem like there's no end to the challenges we face when we try to create the strong, supportive community we know our children need to grow up strong, self-confident, and secure. It can seem like we're out-numbered, out-budgeted, and out-shouted—so we're licked before we start. But that's just not true!

Sure, parents who want to create a healthy lifestyle for their kids have many barriers to overcome, from the incessant junk-food ads to the lure of sedentary activities that lead to a sedentary lifestyle in front of a video screen. And it doesn't help when their local schools offer kiosks of fast-foods in the cafeteria and candy and soft-drinks in vending machines down the halls. Then there's the trend to cut back on gym classes in school and shut down public recreation areas, not to mention dousing the street-lamps, giving our kids fewer and fewer places to play. No doubt about it, it can sometimes seem pretty hopeless.

But we all have the power we need to re-create the kind of community in which our kids can thrive. We just need to take *ACTION!* And if you don't know how to get started, or where to look for allies in achieving this goal, well, just read on—this chapter is devoted to giving you exactly the kind of practical guidance you're looking for.

GETTING STARTED

Step one in creating a better community for your kids is to take an inventory of just what your "dream" community would offer them. That way you can take stock of what's already in place and what's not, and then target your efforts to fill the gaps. In my mind, a healthy community for kids would include the following basic "senses":

- A sense of "neighborhood"—whether that means a suburban street, a country town, or an urban high-rise apartment building—the place that a kid calls home and the people who live nearby are what constitutes a neighborhood. But it takes more than a bunch of nearby people to make such a place feel "neighborly." For *that*, you need to feel that those people know—and care—that you exist.

- A sense of support—in a healthy community, your kids would feel that the people around them are *for and with* them, not against them. In such a community, kids dare to test their limits, indulge their creativity, and even risk failure—they know they can count on the people around them to appreciate their effort, not laugh at them if they fall short of achieving what they set out to do. And because they feel that support, they're more likely to be willing to "try, try again."

- A sense of continuity—in a high-speed, high-stress, and highly mobile world like ours, this is perhaps the most important, and the most difficult value to provide for our kids. But that's exactly why it's more important than ever to give our kids the feeling that there are people and ideals that they can count on. Ideals like the unconditional love of their families and friends, and clear-cut rules and expectations. Sure, kids complain when parents tell them "no" about something they want to have or do—but if your rules are reasonable, and if you're fair about the way you enforce them, you'll discover that kids are actually grateful for them. After all, without rules, life can feel overwhelming and pretty chaotic.

Okay, so how does *your* community measure up in these general areas of concern? If it doesn't stack up very well, right now, don't feel alone. These may be basic issues, but they're pretty hard to address. Still, you don't have to settle for a community that doesn't satisfy these needs. Read on to learn how you can help to create one that *does!*

CREATING A NEIGHBORHOOD

Let's start with the idea that every child needs to feel that there's someplace where he or she truly belongs. That's what a sense of neighborhood provides. And at the core of the neighborhood is... you guessed it, the family. I know I've said this over and over again in this book, but it's true—parents are every child's first role models, and to build a strong relationship, parents and children must spend time together. Lots of things work against us in this area, however—from the lure of the TV and the Internet to the simple fact that our lives are so over-scheduled that it's hard to find time to come together.

On the Family Front

What to do? First and foremost, establish an "at least one meal together" rule, and make it stick. And make certain to set enough time aside for this family meal so that everyone actually has a chance to talk to one another. It doesn't count if everybody at the table has their noses buried in a book, or if the TV is on and you're all munching absent-mindedly while staring, zombie-eyed, at the screen. This mealtime should be spent sharing the news of your day with one another—and even the littlest ones should be made to feel that their contribution is welcome and appreciated. And, of course, mealtime rules should also require that everyone stays at the table until everyone else is finished eating. I've already explained how this helps dysfunctional eaters to slow down and really taste their food, but it also guarantees that everyone has a chance to really talk.

Next, don't give in to the current trend—refuse to give the kids a TV in their own rooms. If you get into the habit of treating TV viewing as a family affair, you reap a *lot* of benefits. First, you have a much better chance to monitor what your kids are watching, which means you can step in and change the channel if you find they're viewing programs that you find objectionable. Second, you have a chance to rebut some of the advertising messages that are designed to hoodwink kids into demanding stuff you *know* is not good for them. Third, the shows you watch together will give you plenty of opportunities to explore how your kids feel about the world and about themselves—since the discussions come up in the context of a TV show, you'll find your kids will feel more free to talk about their feelings without feeling as if you're being intrusive.

For many of the same reasons, don't set up the kids' computers in their bedrooms, at least until they're in high school. The Internet can be a pretty dangerous place for kids—with everything from aggressively e-mailing pornography sites to the sicko's who actually use the kid-oriented chat rooms to prey on our children. If you're unaware of what your kids are up to when they're on-line, you can't protect them. And by all means set some limits about the time they spend on the computer—a 4-hour stint surfing the Internet or tinkering away on a computer game is no substitute for active play.

And there's lots more you can do to create a strong sense of family. For example, you can make a point of setting some time aside each weekend for kid-oriented activities, and whenever possible, you'll want to schedule activities that also contribute to fitness. In nice weather, a picnic plus a family game or sport—even something as simple as tossing a Frisbee around can be a lot of fun for everybody. For those who live in colder climate zones, winter can mean an occasional family snowball fight or skating party. You get the idea, right? Or, if your kids participate in a formal sports team, make a point of at least attending the major games as a family, so you can all cheer your young athlete on. Believe me, even kids who avoid acknowledging their parents, for fear of looking dorky to their pals, are secretly pleased to know that the family cares enough to show up for "the big game."

See—it's not that hard to build family possibilities into your days. All you have to do is make the commitment.

Neighborhood Beyond the Family

A strong sense of family is essential to helping children develop confidence and self-esteem, but it's also important to create a larger world in which they feel like they belong. Here, too, you have to take the lead—if you resist making connections with the people who live and work near you, it can't come as a surprise that your child will also feel isolated or even alienated.

Here, too, the practical steps you can take are pretty basic. Make a point of making eye-contact with your neighbors, whether you run into them on the suburban street where you live, or share an elevator up to your big-city apartment. Share an observation about the day's weather with the clerk who rings up your groceries, at your regular supermarket or the local deli. *Smile.* Sure, some people will refuse to respond, but most people are like you—looking for a way to make connections in their neighborhood. And once you've cracked the ice, you'll have begun building a collection of people who don't just live and work nearby—they actually form a neighborhood.

As you build relationships with your neighbors, your family, and especially your children, find a larger world in which they are known, at least by name and by sight. They also learn to dare to be a little more outgoing, simply by observing your good example. At the same time, you can use this as an opportunity to teach valuable lessons about safety—explaining why it's okay to talk to neighborhood "regulars" but not to strangers, for example.

Out on Their Own

Neighborhood and community extends even further than this, however—to places where parents are frequently, even usually, absent. School is a prime example of this. Here, too, however, you can actively build a strong sense of community—and your efforts will be more than welcome.

For example, most teachers are seriously distressed by how few parents get involved in their kids' school lives. On parent-teacher nights, the hallways are often empty, and the teachers wait in vain for a few parents to turn up to discuss their kids' progress. How can you convince your child that their school-work is important, if you don't show up on those few important nights each year?

Kids in the lower grades commonly spend a great deal of time working on projects to be displayed to their parents—and it really *does* mean more to them if you see the proud results of their finger-painting on the display board in the classroom than if you wait until they're allowed to bring it home. Older kids may be less obvious about it, but even they notice if you don't go to see their teachers—and that's just as true for the kids who are having trouble in school as it is for the ones who know you're going to hear only good reports.

And there's another reason why your attendance at school functions really matters—it gives you more influence if you want to change school policies that you disagree with. Parents who become known to the school administrators are more likely to be listened to when they raise concerns—such as protesting the quality of the school lunch, the installation of fast-food kiosks and vending machines in the cafeteria, or by proposing an after-school program.

Outside of school, you can also create a sense of neighbor-hood in the world of your child's friends, even though you may not always be around when they're playing together. You do this sim-ply by making a point of getting to know the other parents. Oddly enough, a lot of parents make a point of getting to know little Susie or Joey's friends, but never think of picking up the phone and in-troducing themselves to the parents of their friends houses. Yet, if your children are playing together, they're probably spending some time in each other's homes—so doesn't it make sense for the parents to get to know each other, at least a little? How else can you know whether or not your child is being exposed to influences that suit your values?

Believe it or not, this is at least as important for your older children as it is for your little ones. And even when kids complain about their parents "butting in" this way, they're usually pretty glad to know that you care enough to make the effort to look out for their interests. And who knows, as an added benefit, you just may end up making a new friend or two yourself!

CREATING A SUPPORTIVE UNIVERSE

A sense of support is next on our list of basic values. Much of the work required to give your children the feeling that they are supported by their community will be done simply by taking the steps outlined above for creating a "neighborhood." After all, those steps are primarily designed to build communication in the home and expand the "outside" network of people that your child knows he or she can trust, because you have come to trust them. But there's a lot more you can do, too.

Talking to Our Children

For instance, you can pay close attention to the words you use when speaking with your child. Are you prone to using "you" language—the kind of thing that comes across as commands and accusations? Or are you more likely to use "I" language—in which you share your concerns or feelings about things? Do you often feel like a 'broken record,' spending more time finding fault than offering honest praise?

Kids take what we say very much to heart, and a sharp word that feels unfairly delivered can be like a stab to the heart. That doesn't mean you can't correct a child—it simply means that we must pay very close attention to how our words are heard.

Very often, well-meaning parents who hope to encourage their children to succeed (and even excel) will withhold praise along the way, giving it only after some major goal has been achieved. But it's hard for kids—especially very young kids—to keep up a sustained effort in a vacuum. Encouragement along the way, for even the smallest feat, is *greatly* appreciated. In this way they're not much different than adults—how often have *you* felt unappreciated at work because your boss never seems to notice your everyday efforts, and only speaks up when you make a mistake?

But remember—what kids need is encouragement, not bribes! What they really need is your honest appreciation, not rewards of food or toys or cash. Too often, parents hand out prizes instead of the one thing kids want most—attention and emotional approval.

A Safety Network

Most parents today can't manage to *be there* for their kids, even if they truly want to. So many of us are trying to manage homes with 2 working parents, and so many others are trying to juggle our jobs and single parenthood. But kids need to feel safe and supported all the time, not just when we're free of our other obligations.

This can be one of the most difficult challenges we face in creating a healthy community, especially if we have no family living nearby. But even here there are things we can do to expand our children's sense of community. Here are some suggestions:

- Form alliances with other parents. Since the problem is so widespread, just about every other parent you meet is probably dealing with it to. Talk to the other parents on your street or in your building, and look for a few with whom you would feel comfortable in setting up a sort of "time-share" relationship. Then you can take turns hosting each other's kids a few days each week, so each of you has a few days off in which to take care of other obligations, but you can rest assured knowing that your child is in good hands. Think of it as a variation on the car-pooling theme and you've got the idea.

- Explore possibilities at your workplace. Many employers —but not yet nearly enough of them—now offer on-premises child-care services. Many others are willing to accept the reality of to-day's life—that there are times when work schedules don't exactly mesh with school or daycare schedules—and permit parents to work from home or to bring their kids to work on those occasions when no other solution is available. If your employer is not yet one of these enlightened beings, consider bringing the issue up with your boss or the company's human resources department. (Hint: it's best to bring it up with at least 2 or 3 other employees who have children.)

- Talk to your children's school administrators or your childcare provider about the possibility of "off-hours" activities for children. I'm not just talking about after- hours care here, I mean *real activities*—not a place where the kids watch videos or play computer games. There may be an after-school program in place for children whose parents can't be home when school is out, for example. Or if there is no such program but the need for it is clear, you might be able to get one started. Similarly, some childcare providers are willing to extend their hours on occasion or for an additional fee—but you won't know unless you ask!

- Check out community-based options. The "local government" pages of your phone book is a good place to start. For example, lots of local libraries sponsor an after-school story-hour for kids, and many communities have an active "cultural affairs" department, usually included under "Human Services" that sponsors kid-oriented activities. If you're wired to the "Net," you can check your city or state Website—even the smallest communities have gone on-line with information about local resources, these days.

Whatever you do, make a point of having people lined up to serve as "back-up" in case of emergencies—and make sure your children know who these people are. There's nothing scarier to kids—of *any* age—than to think that they've been forgotten.

CREATING CONTINUITY

Creating continuity can be tricky, too—especially since our society has become so mobile. Divorce, job transfers, and other pressures all contribute to a child's sense that there's no place to put down roots. We can't turn back the clock to a simpler time when people stayed in the same community for generations on end, but we *can* make an effort to create a sense of stability, none-theless. It just takes a little more effort.

Perhaps the most effective way to give our children a sense of stability and continuity is by providing consistency in the rules and values we set forth for them. If a child grows up knowing that these are unchanging, their very predictability provides a sense of comfort. I'm not here to preach my values and beliefs to you and encourage you to adopt them all for your own kids, because these are things that each of you as parents must work out for yourself. What matters most of all is that the rules we establish are fair, consistently applied, and clearly ex-plained—to the degree appropriate to our children's ages.

That last point is important. Kids don't need to have the power to write the rules, but they do deserve to be told why the rules exist in the first place. Think back to your own childhood and you'll probably remember times when you felt things were terribly unjust—and you'll probably also remember that those were the times when the answer to your question "why?" was a bland "because I said so!" Kids have a powerful sense of injustice, but they are also very receptive to reason.

The trick is to be willing to provide explanations appropriate to your child's age and development, without opening every rule up to wrangling and bargaining. After all, *you* are the parent. If your rules are reasonable and in your children's best interest, you don't need to get defensive when they're challenged—you simply explain the reasoning behind them and move on. End of discussion!

WORKING IN THE WIDER WORLD

Creating and maintaining a set of values that help your children develop a strong sense of self-esteem and self-confidence will go a long way toward insulating them from some of the outside pressures we discussed earlier in this book: everything from peer pressure to the media onslaught. But that's not your only line of defense. If you've got the time and the ability, there are many ways you can get active in the effort to reverse some of today's more damaging trends. Let's take a look at a few areas where you can turn your commitment to building a healthy lifestyle for your family into some truly effective activism.

Reversing School Policy Trends

By now you should be pretty well aware that I've got a few complaints to make about how our public officials have basically extinguished our schools' physical education programs. And you've probably noticed that I'm appalled by the trend of installing fast-food kiosks and junk-food vending machines in the cafeterias, of teachers using food as rewards for class work, and other such erroneous policy decisions. The thing to keep in mind is that these decisions aren't irreversible. As a member of the community, and particularly as a parent, you have every right to make your voice heard. The question is, how can you make your voice heard *effectively*.

Step one is to get to know your school board. Your phone book has a listing for the board that operates in your school district, and you can contact that office to request a list of the board members. Your local paper is another important resource—it will publish the dates of school board meetings and notify you when meetings are open to the public. Pay attention to how individual board members vote in decisions that concern you. In most communities, these people are elected—and if you don't like their decisions, you can work to *un*-elect them.

Step two is to talk to other parents. If you find that a substantial number of them share your views, you can form a group to bring your concerns to the attention of your school administration and your school board. There's strength in numbers—and you just may find that there are many people out there who were just *waiting* for someone to take the lead.

Even if you don't succeed in getting official policy changed—for example, if you're trying to get an after-school activity program installed, you might find other creative ways to achieve your goal. For instance, if your school board won't officially establish the program, you might find them willing to allow a parent-run program to be offered on school grounds, if you've taken steps to get one organized.

Another area where you can work effectively is to improve the nutritional content of the food served in the school cafeteria. All public schools are required to serve food that meets certain nutritional standards, which are available for viewing on the USDA Website. Check out your school's lunch offerings—and enlist the help of some of the other parents if you must. If you feel that your school is falling short, you have every right to raise the issue with your school's administration. And if that isn't enough, you can take it up with the school board.

Fighting the Media Blitz

Reversing the damaging anti-health, anti-self-esteem, anti-anything-valuable-to-our-self-worth messages of the media is perhaps the toughest problem of all. There are just so many profits to be made by corporations who push unhealthy products on an unwary public. That's why many of them use the promise of "fund raising" to communities and institutions in need of funds—like our schools, which are always looking for extra sources of funds now that budgets have been cut so badly. Well, one thing we're all learning is that this corporate "free money" isn't really free at all—it's given to schools and institutions in return for access to our children!

Your best defense against media manipulation is to become aware of it whenever and wherever it appears—and when you spot something that offends you, vote with your pocketbook! Don't buy products made by the offending corporation. And the best way to protect your children from this same manipulation is to begin educating them *early*! That means refusing to let the half-truths and even outright misrepresentation go unchallenged. Here's how:

- Watch TV with your kids, and talk to them about the commercials that seem to run every couple of minutes on child-oriented programs.

- Make a game out of "spotting the falsehoods." As I mentioned earlier, kids just *love* to feel that they've seen through a trick—especially if the "tricker" is a grown-up.

- Get your kids actively involved in a little "counter- programming." This one can be a lot of fun, and just might unleash a little creativity in your kids. For example, instead of caving in and providing the highly advertised, brand- name sodas, offer a home-made water-and-juice or seltzer-and-juice concoction, and challenge the kids to come up with your *own* "advertising" slogan or jingle.

A BETTER FUTURE

For our kid's sake—and for our own—there's nothing more important than encouraging the development of strong, self-confident children. They are, after all, our future. The sad thing is that many parents seem to have lost sight of how wonderfully rewarding this can be. In the rush and bustle of modern life, we can easily forget that the precious moments of childhood just *fly* by—and when we miss a milestone in our children's lives, it's an opportunity that simply won't come again. The rewards that come from raising happy, healthy children are very great, and outweigh any materialistic goals we can ever try to achieve.

So, let's work together to give our children a life of *food, fun, n' fitness.* We'll all be the richer for it!

Appendix A:
Children's Bill of Rights

- All children should be assured of healthy minds & healthy bodies
- All children should be protected against abuse and neglect and other harmful treatment
- All children who have special mental or physical needs should be provided with an appropriate education and medical care
- All children should be provided with adequate nourishment, housing and clothing
- All children should have access to wholesome recreational and cultural resources
- All children should be protected against disease and injury
- All children should be educated in accordance with their capacities
- All preschool children should be provided with a safe, stimulating environment in which they can achieve school readiness
- All children should be given a sense of family and community so that they can become productive members of society
- All children should be given due regard as members of our society

(Created by the Children's Services Council of Palm Beach County and the Child Advocacy Board of Palm Beach County, Florida.)

Appendix B:
Further Resources

- American Psychiatric Association. *Diagnostic and Statistical Manual of Mental Disorders*. Fourth ed. Washington, DC: American Psychiatric Association, 1994.
- Barnette, Martha. "Tech Toys: How Are They Really Affecting Your Child?" *Child* (February 2001): 92–95.
- Berg, Frances M. *Afraid To Eat: Children and Teens in Weight Crisis*. Healthy Weight Journal Publications, 1997.
    - "Why Teenage Girls Drop Out of Sports." *Healthy Weight Journal* 8 (1994): 1–13.
- Bruch, Hilde. *Eating Disorders: Obesity, Anorexia Nervosa, and the Person Within*. New York: Basic Books, 1973.
- Cohen, Cathi. "Teaching Skills for Social Stress." Washington Parent: www.family2go.com/raisingkids/child/skills/features/family_1998_05/dcpt58stress.htm
- Cooper, Kenneth H. *Fit Kids! The Complete Shape-Up Program from Birth through High School*. Nashville, TN: Broadman and Holman, Publishers, 1999.
- Cloud, John. "The Goddess of Go-Gurt." *Time* (November 13, 2000).
- Dean, Carolyn. "Sweet Conspiracy." *Natural Health* (January/February 2001): 74–79, 124–125.
- Evitt, Marie Faust. "Could Your Praise be Hurting Your Child?" *Child* (November 2000): 100–104.
- Hall, Ross Hume. *The Unofficial Guide to Smart Nutrition*. New York: IDG Books, Worldwide. 2000.
- Katch, Frank, and William McArdle. *Introduction to Nutrition, Exercise, and Health*. Philadelphia: Lee and Febiger, 1993
- Kushner, Rabbi Harold S. "Nourishing Your Child's Soul." *Child* (December/January 2000/2001): 61–64.
- Leach, Penelope. *Babyhood*. Second edition. New York: Knopf, 2000.

- Lemonick, Michael D. "Teens before Their Time." *Time* (October 30, 2000).
- McCarthy, Laura Flynn. "Raising a Stress-Free Child." *Parenting* (March 2001): 66–70.
- Michaud, Ellen. "Reconnect." *Prevention* (December 2000): 122–129.
- Omichinski, Linda, and K. R. Harrison. *Weight Management for Teens: A Non-diet Approach to Health and Fitness for Adolescents.* San Marcos, CA: Nutrition Dimension, 1997.
- Pierre, Colleen. "Is Sugar Making You Fat?" *Prevention* (January 2001): 118–125.
- "The Salt Treaty." *Child* (November 2000): 43–47.
- Poussant, Alvin, and Susan Linn. "Surviving Television Advertising." Family Education Network: www.familyeducation.com/article/0,1120,3-1528,00.html?oe8
- Povis Alleman, Gayle. *Save Your Child from the Fat Epidemic: 7 Steps Every Parent Can Take to Ensure Healthy, Fit Children for Life.* Rocklin, CA: Prima Publishing.
- Queen, P. M., and C. E. Lang, eds. *Handbook of Pediatric Nutrition.* Gaithersberg, MD: Aspen Publishers, 1993.
- Roosevelt, Margot. "A Spoonful of Sugar? Beware." *Time* (November 13, 2000): 95.
- Schlosser, Eric. *Fast Food Nation: The Dark Side of the All-American Meal.* New York: Houghton-Mifflin, 2001.
- Schultz, Susan. "The Missing Fitness Link." *Shape* (January 2001): 110–117.
- Steen, Suzanne. *Nutrition for Young Athletes.* San Marcos, CA: Nutrition Dimension, Inc., 1994.
- Strong, William B, and Jack H Wilmore. "Unfit Kids: An Office-Based Approach to Physical Fitness." *Contemporary Pediatrics* (April 1988): 34.
- Steward, H. Leighton, Morrison C. Bethea, Sam S. Andrews, and Luis A. Balart. *Sugar Busters! Cut Sugar to Trim Fat.* New York: Ballantine Publishing, 1998.
- U.S. Department of Agriculture, Human Nutrition Services. "Food Guide Pyramid: A Guide to Daily Food Choices." *Home and Garden Bulletin No. 252.* Washington, D.C.: Government Printing Office.

Internet Resources

General Health and Nutrition

- About Nutrition. About.com Web site devoted to nutrition issues. www.nutrition.about.com
- American Academy of Pediatrics: www.aap.org
- American Diabetes Association: www.diabetes.org
- American Dietetic Association: www.eatright.org
- American Heart Association: www.americanheart.org
- Arbor Nutrition Guide: http://arborcom.com
- Centers for Disease Control and Prevention: www.cdc.gov
- Center for Science in the Public Interest (CSPI): www.cspinet.org
- Cyberdiet. Web site devoted to health and nutrition. www.cyberdiet.com
- Discovery Health. A Web site sponsored by the Discovery Network: www.discoveryhealth.com
- KidsHealth. Website on childhood wellness issues sponsored by the Nemours Foundation: www.kidshealth.org
- National Cancer Institute): www.5aday.gov
- National Osteoporosis Foundation: www.NOF.org
- Tufts' Navigator: navigator.tufts.edu
- WebMD: www.webmd.com

Physical Activity and Exercise

- American College of Sports Medicine: www.acsm.org
- American Council on Exercise: www.acefitness.com
- GirlPower! A web page of the U.S. Department of Health and Human Services: www.health.org/gpower
- International Life Sciences Institute (ILSI). Information on school fitness activities programs: www.ilsi.org
- SPARK (sports, play, and active recreation for kids): send email to sparkpe@mail.sdsu.edu

Obesity and Eating Disorders

- American Anorexia Bulimia Association: www.aabainc.org
- Committed to Kids Pediatric Weight Management Program (developed in conjunction with Louisiana State University: www.committed-to-kids.com
- Eating Disorders Awareness and Prevention, Inc.: www.edap.org
- National Association of Anorexia Nervosa and Associated Eating Disorders: www.anad.org
- National Eating Disorders Organization (NEDO): www.laureate.com
- National Institutes of Health Weight Control Information Network (WIN): www.niddk.nih.gov/health/nutri/win.htm
- Overeaters Anonymous: www.overeatersanonymous.org
- Shape Up America! (headed by former surgeon general C. Everett Koop): www.shapeup.org

Healthy-Cooking Websites

- www.cookinglight.com
- www.cookingwithkids.com
- www.epicurious.com
- www.familyfoodzone.com/cooking
- www.kitchenlink.com
- www.planetveggie.com
- www.scoreone.com/kids_kitchen
- www.vegetariantimes.com

Kids and Teens

- Center for the Advancement of Children's Mental Health: www.kidsmentalhealth.org
- TV Turnoff Network: www.tvturnoff.org
- Center for Commercial-Free Public Education: www.commercialfree.org
- Centers for Disease Control School Health Index: www.cdc.gov/nccdphp/dash

- National Association for Girls and Women in Sport: www.aahperd.org
- National Dairy Council Interactive Kids Zone: www.nutritionexplorations.org
- Smart Girl (self esteem issues): www.smartgirl.com

Resource Kits

- From the National Heart, Lung, and Blood Institute (a division of the National Institutes of Health: CATCH (child and adolescent trial for cardiovascular health) and GO-FOR-HEALTH; : a Nationally tested school-based programs. Write to the NHLBI Info Center at P.O Box 30105, Bethesda, MD 20824-0105.
- NHLBI and the National Recreation and Park Association (NRPA): Hearts & Parks Jump Start. Write to the NRPA at 22377 Belmont Ridge Road, Ashburn, VA 20148.
- Project Fit America: working with schools to support fitness programs. Write to the project at 760 Market Street #907, San Francisco, CA 94102.
- School Food Service Foundation of the American School Food Service Association: *Healthy EDGE 2000, The Dietary Guidelines and Education.* Write for information to the Food Service Foundation, American Food Service Association, 1600 Duke Street, 7th Floor, Alexandria, VA 22314-3436.
- USDA Bureau of Food and Nutrition, Department of Education: Team Nutrition modules for pre-K through 8th grade. Write to the Bureau of Food and Nutrition, Dept. of Ed., Grimes State Office Building, Des Moines, IA 50319.

Vegetarian Sites

- Soyfoods Association of America, One Sutter Street, Suite 300, San Francisco, CA 94104.
- United Soybean Board, Soy Hotline: 1-800-TALK-SOY
- Vegetarian Resource Group: www.vgr.org
- Vegetarian Times: www.vegetariantimes.com

Index

About the Author

Mary C. Friesz, PhD, RD, CDE, LDN, received her B.S. degree in nutrition from the University of Massachusetts at Amherst in 1986, her M.S. in both nutrition and exercise physiology from Columbia University's Teacher's College in 1989, and her Ph.D. from Monticello University in 1999. She fulfilled her dietetic internship at Columbia Presbyterian Medical Center in New York in 1990, was accredited as a registered dietician by the American Dietetic Association in 1991 and is a Licensed Dietician in the state of Florida. She was certified as a Certified Diabetes Educator by the National Certification Board for Diabetes Educators in 1992. She was accredited as a Certified Aerobic and Exercise Instructor by the American Council on Exercise in 1988.

Mary is a member of the American Dietetic Association, the American Diabetes Association, the Broward County Dietetic Association, the Palm Beach County Dietetic Association, the American Council on Exercise, and the South Florida Association of Diabetes Educators. She has been in private practice as a nutrition and wellness consultant since 1987.

Mary has devoted much her career to providing professional lifestyle counseling and nutrition and fitness guidance to individuals suffering from obesity and eating disorders, and she brings a special sensitivity to these issues because she knows, first-hand, what her clients are going through. She has spent more than 15 years in clinical practice, bringing her unique blend of professional training and personal empathy to the care of her clients. To bring her message to a broader audience, Mary also maintains a popular website, at www.designs4health.com, where she offers regular topical articles of interest to consumers, and advice for colleagues in the health service professions.

To order additional copies of this book, you can order it online at www.foodfunnfitness.com. or use the handy coupon on the next page to order by fax or mail.

Name_____

Address _____

City_____State____Zip _____

Phone _____

E-Mail address_____

# of Books at $14.95 _____ + $3.00 S&H.:

Total:_____ (*FL residents add 6% sales tax)

Method of Payment:

Check_____ Visa _____ MasterCard___ Am Ex ____Novus_____

Credit Card Number_____

Security Code (3 or 4 digit # on front of card (back on Am Ex)____

Credit Card Expiration Date_____

Name as it appears on card _____

Signature _____

To order by fax, send to 561-999-0863

To order by mail, send to: _____

    Mary C. Friesz, PhD, RD, CDE, LDN
    Attn: Food, Fun n' Fitness
    P.O. Box 81-1974
    Boca Raton, FL 33481-1974

    *Bulk Order Discounts:
    10-24 books = 25% off
    25+ = 35% off

*For more information about using "Food Fun n Fitness" for your next fund-raiser, please call Dr. Mary at 561-999-8941 or 954-370-9278.